Healing Our Backs with Yoga

An Essential Guide to Back Pain Relief

by Lillah A. Schwartz

Published by Beneficial Services Inc. through Ingram Press

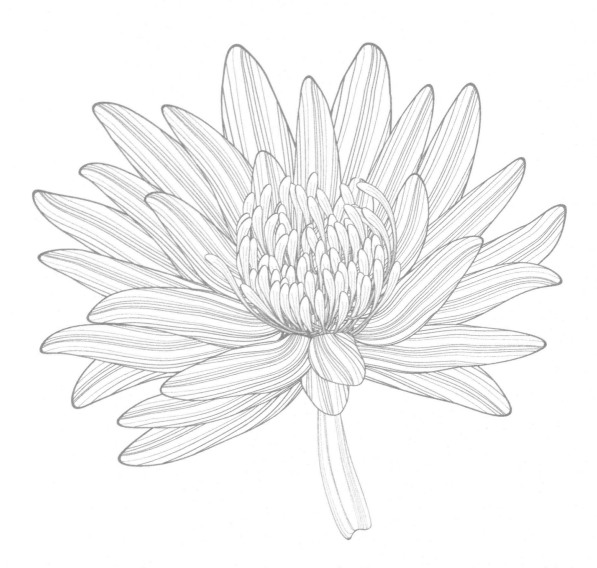

Published by Beneficial Services Inc. through Ingram Press
All images and text ©Lillah Schwartz 2016, unless otherwise specified.

Available for order through Ingram Press Catalogues or directly from the author.
Lillah Albano Schwartz

Digital copies avaialble at
www.YogawithLillah.com
www.LillahSchwartz.com

Printed in the United States of America
First Printing June 2016
Published by Beneficial Services Inc.

ISBN: 978-0-9643835-5-5

Table of Contents

Acknowledgements

I dedicate this book with my deepest gratitude to B.K.S. Iyengar. The vision and skill he shared were the fountain of wisdom that shaped the understanding and skill I offer my students today. And to my yoga mentors Felicity Green and Eric Small for the ways they have enhanced my understanding.

Thank you also to:

- My beloved husband, Gary, without whom none of this would have been possible;
- All my teachers along the healing path too numerous to mention;
- My students who have challenged, inspired, and blessed me with their need, responsiveness, and dedication to their own healing with yoga;
- My friend and fellow healer Catherine Carrigan for her priceless encouragement;
- Maggie Powell who orchestrated the layout of this book so beautifully;
- And the other people who offered counsel and moral support, including Michelle Van Sandt and Angie Young for their photography and photoshop skills; and Becky Shipkowsky who helped me understand the consistency and details needed to write a book;
- To all of my beloved students who modeled for photographs; Jennifer Phelps, Stacy Stone, Ann Mundy, Mili Perez, Letitia Walker, Anna Roques;
- And last but not least, my editor, Deborah Morgenthal, who made me sound like an English major!

The blessings offered though yoga never end. May my humble offerings in this book be a blessing to you on your healing journey.

Disclaimer: Choose Safety

This book is designed to help those with pain from muscular-skeletal back and neck conditions, spinal arthritis, osteoporosis, sacroiliac joint dysfunction, spinal disc bulges or herniations, and mild scoliosis.

There are back conditions that are beyond the scope of this book, such as spinal stenosis that creates consistent numbness in the limbs, conditions of inflammation like rheumatoid arthritis, or conditions where neurological damage is a limiting factor such as Multiple Sclerosis and Parkinson's. In general, if you're experiencing a high level of back pain above a 5 on a scale of 1 to 10, please consult with your health care professional before beginning this or any other exercise program.

The information in this book is not a substitute for medical treatment. Please consult with your healthcare professional:

+ If you experience a worsening in severity or duration of your pain after you begin the sequences presented.
+ If one or both legs or arms develop weakness or numbness when you practice the sequences.
+ If you experience any other odd symptoms as a result of your practice.

If you're recovering from a surgery, including back, shoulder, hip, or knee replacement, please wait until you have full clearance from your doctor and physical therapist before beginning this program.

Learn as much as you can about your particular condition. Knowledge is power and will help you apply the principles that will be presented here.

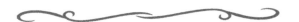

Foreword

by Catherine Carrigan

Like many of Lillah Schwartz's new yoga students, I had injured myself before I began studying and practicing with her. I had ripped the tendons and ligaments in my right shoulder through a series of unfortunate accidents. My right shoulder hurt so badly it was difficult to pick up my purse or walk my dog on a leash. Although I had practiced and taught yoga for 18 years at that point, I was not able to do a single down dog. Chatturanga was simply out of the question. Headstand, wheel, shoulderstand, forearm stand—these familiar poses felt like they were quickly about to become part of my past.

On top of the physical injury, I had gone through two years of unremitting life traumas, one right after the other with no pause to recover. I knew I needed to practice as much yoga as possible to repair my shoulder and restore my soul. That's what brought me to the master healer Lillah Schwartz.

While rebalancing my shoulder in her class, I had the privilege of observing Lillah work her magic on every manner of serious structural injury—neck pain, shoulder pain, back pain, hip pain, knee pain, foot pain. As a medical intuitive healer myself, I was delighted to discover myself in the company of a powerful woman who kindly guided regular folks—many of whom had never practiced yoga before—from suffering to inner peace.

After studying with Lillah, I was delighted to discover that I too could guide an injured person from agony to relief by showing them a short yoga sequence. If you have been suffering, please pay close attention. Many may hope to heal you, but it's the true master teacher who can actually deliver on her good intentions.

Lillah Schwartz is the master teacher you have been searching and possibly praying for.

I am thankful that my injured shoulder led me to Lillah and grateful for all the wisdom she generously shares in this wonderful book that you now hold in your hands.

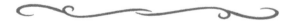

Catherine Carrigan is a medical intuitive healer and four-time Amazon No. 1 Best Selling Author of *What Is Healing?*, *Awaken Your Intuitive Power for Health, Happiness and Unlimited Energy Now*, *Banish the Blues*, and *Unlimited Intuition NOW*. She integrates the very best in fitness, nutrition, and natural healing to empower you to achieve exceptional levels of health and well-being.

Message from the Author

When I started teaching yoga for back care in 1987, the therapeutic benefits of yoga were largely unknown. Today, with so many new teachers and practitioners, people have a better idea of what yoga has to offer. Still, the understanding of it as a therapeutic art is relatively new.

The training and approach to yoga I share follow the alignment principles of a world-renowned yoga master, B.K.S. Iyengar. Mr. Iyengar's methods were developed primarily from a subjective, experiential, and intuitive platform, yet they are substantiated by the principles of anatomy, physiology, and kinesiology. In some ways, Iyengar yoga practiced as a healing art moves even beyond modalities, such as physical therapy, sports medicine, and Rolfing. According to this method, the practice of yoga is an integrative art, moving students toward longer-lasting pain relief, renewed self-confidence, and a sense of wholeness.

In life, there are a variety of reasons that back, neck, or shoulder pain may arise, including a fall or other accident, poor posture, repetitive motion, chronic tension from stress and overuse, or lack of flexibility. Consider a person who performs the same activity over many years, such as tennis, golf, computer work, sewing, hiking, etc. Repeated use without stretching causes muscles to shorten and become rigid. Eventually, such rigidity leads to degeneration inside the joint that has lost its movement, with corresponding wear and tear in the more moveable joints used to compensate for the lack of movement elsewhere. A good yoga program to counterbalance these activities—as a preventative and /or postural corrective measure—could easily and effectively be put in place. So whether you are new to yoga, a regular practitioner, or a yoga teacher, I believe the ideas and suggestions in these pages will guide your yoga practice and healing journey.

This book is the culmination of my 33 years studying physical sciences, practicing and teaching yoga, and working with countless students and clients who suffered from back, neck, and shoulder pain. The principles of yoga and movement I share in this book are time tested and reliable. Therefore, if you're looking to heal or prevent back pain issues and improve spinal health and vitality, this book is for you. By becoming knowledgeable about the principles offered here, you can open the door to healing and self-discovery.

Yoga itself is a vast art that takes years to master. The motivation behind this book is to offer you an understanding of yoga that is simple, direct, and easy to apply in order that you find your way to greater ease, hopefully avoiding surgery and the continued discomfort of back pain.

Remember that our bodies are like clay and will take on any shape according to the pattern of movement we do most frequently. A yoga practice offers ideal movement choices for remolding our bodies to create better balance, relieve pain, and prevent future discomfort.

Please accept my seasoned offerings, and may our lives continue to be blessed by Yoga.

Sincerely, Lillah

Is This Book For You?

As I mentioned in my message, our bodies are like clay: they mold themselves into the form of whatever activity we perform on a regular basis. Consequently, sitting at the computer all day, or being engaged in any activity where we sit for long hours, as well as other repeated activities that we do either for work or pleasure, will have their effect. The idea for someone who is looking for back pain relief is to find yoga poses that counterbalance those activities and postures, and then practice them on a regular basis. Regularity is the key.

Bodywork professionals such as Physiatrists, Rolfers, massage therapists, physical therapists, and personal trainers know well that the body heals itself through movement. Therefore, the right movement, exercise, or yoga pose for the right problem mobilizes the body's healing force with resulting improvement in function.

Anyone beginning a yoga journey and practice is confronted by the challenge of creating a more comprehensive mind-body relationship. Even though we live in our bodies, we are often disconnected from them, living more in our mental image of who we are, rather than connecting to the more subtle messages from our various parts. When something goes wrong, such as the sudden appearance of back pain, we assume our bodies are broken and we have no idea how it happened. The truth is that the imbalance and injury may have been happening for five, ten, or maybe twenty years—maybe even as a result of our yoga practice. We simply did not have the tools or understanding to interpret the messages of the body to avoid the future discomfort we are currently faced with.

My experience over the years as a yoga teacher has convinced me that when people take the time to learn the basics of anatomy, posture, and alignment, and come to understand how to apply the fundamental movement principles to their particular condition, they can more successfully manage and support their own healing process and journey to pain relief.

Those of you who are already a student or a teacher of yoga may also find yourself experiencing back pain. Your yoga practice may have given you relief in the beginning; however, the discomfort may linger or grow worse with the way you're practicing, making lasting relief illusive. You may even begin to consider that you're damaged, or simply getting old. Perish the thought! I suspect that some fundamental alignment and movement principles are missing from your understanding. The approach I offer here is a way to re-think and re-apply the principles of alignment, action, and breath to your asana practice.

Yoga is indeed a vast subject, as it takes into account the full gestalt of the human experience and spiritual evolution. Therefore, if your body is calling, it's time to listen and go deeper by acquiring the information and guidance you need to heal your body to create your living temple.

In this book you'll discover ways to apply yoga that are reliable and insightful, and gain new perspectives leading you to a more profound and well-rounded understanding of the application of asana to relieve back, neck, and shoulder pain.

Back pain calls us to spend time with ourselves and our bodies—to learn to move, stretch, and tone in more informed, balanced, and correct ways. Join the many others who have learned to make friends with their bodies and find pain relief.

How to Use This Book

If you have lower back pain, you are not alone. About 80 percent of adults experience low back pain at some point in their lifetimes. However eager you are to begin the yoga program outlined in this book, please refrain from skipping directly to the exercise chapters. The information and insight you'll gain from the preliminary information will open you to new ways of understanding your body, crucial to your success with yoga.

My hope is that this book will create a similar experience of learning that you would gain by attending a therapeutic yoga class with a teacher experienced in helping with back conditions. In the beginning, when we're new to a yoga pose or to the practice of yoga as a healing art, only some awareness is available to our conscious mind. We are able to access the broader actions of each pose, yet the more subtle actions elude us. With practice over time, we become more familiar with the poses, as well as with our bodies and how they respond, and then we're able to have access to and refine our movements for better results and more satisfaction.

Students often worry that they're not doing the poses correctly; they simply cannot yet interpret the feelings they have in order to know they're on the right path. The challenge in yoga then is to learn to listen and feel by practicing the connection of the mind to the breath and the breath to the body so you can uncover your own inner wisdom and discrimination on the path to healing.

I suggest you go through this book systematically, study the background information, the principles of alignment, and then learn the poses in the order suggested. The information presented is essential for you to understand your body in order to positively affect your back health.

You'll notice as you go through the various sequences in this book how some instructions are repeated to remind you to continually reestablish your alignment and use the actions appropriate for the success of each pose and to ensure your safety. This is important: please, pay attention to these reminders.

All the sequences have been created based on the knowledge of functional anatomy and alignment, and tested over time with hundreds of my students to bring you, along with your attention and focus, the best possible experience of ease and balance at their completion. As the book progresses, you'll be lead on a path of improved mobility and function through the addition of new sequences, some new poses, and alternative ways to do basic poses in order for you to fully claim the healing and vitality you desire.

Part 1: Self-Applied Back Care

The book is divided into three sections. The first section, Self-applied Back Care, will provide you with the information necessary to understand how your body works and how to begin your healing journey. So if you're new to yoga, or are someone with back pain that may have lingered after trying other therapies, begin with section number one. The goals for this section are to:

1. Minimize any current pain.
2. Help to create better structural alignment and relative muscular balance.
3. Improve your functional ability.

Before beginning a yoga practice, it's critical to first identify your pain levels: 1 represents no pain, while 10 requires a call to 911. If you're experiencing back pain in the 7 to 10 range, this is an indicator of high levels of inflammation, which is your body's way of protecting you, forcing you to stop and rest. Definitely call your health care professional. Students often come to a back care yoga class with pain levels of 5, 6, or 7 and find relief with the practice, but when you're working on your own, please proceed with caution and use lots of slow deep breathing at that level. Approach your back pain with a beginner's mind, suspend judgment, and observe. Access your pain level objectively using a scale of 1–10 before and after each practice.

Start with the first sequence and repeat it three to five times before moving onto the next sequence. Notice if your pain levels diminish. Continue to practice and work with all the information and sequences from Part 1 until your pain scale is reduced from a level 5–7 to a level 1–3. This could take anywhere from one to three months of regular practice, depending on the severity of your condition. You can then feel confident to move onto the next section.

As a part of this section, you'll be introduced to six basic restorative poses that you can employ at any time during your week to relax and de-stress with the help of more passive yoga poses. Also, you'll be introduced to the magic of Pranayama—yogic breathing—to enhance the depth of your mind-body connection.

Part 2: Building Range of Motion and Strength

As helpful as the basic low back and shoulder sequences are, it's important to move forward in our practice to improve overall flexibility and strength. By increasing our agility and strength, we lessen the risk of back pain in the future. Also, in expanding your practice with this section, you'll discover the greatest change in your posture and vitality levels.

Again the sequences are to be practiced in the order presented for optimal results, repeating each sequence more than once before moving onto the next. Also, intersprecing the sequences from this section with the sequences from part 1 are recommended for optimal ease and balance. Please notice that when a sequence is particularly long, I have included a selection of ways to shorten the sequence to help you maintain your practice when time is limited.

Mastering the sequences and practice guidance given in Parts 1 and 2 will assist you in maintaining good posture and a healthy spine while avoiding those yoga poses that might compromise your safety. Success in yoga is not measured by how many advanced poses you can do, but rather by the amount of awareness and intelligence you apply to the poses you do practice. When back pain relief and back health are your goals, it's better to limit the poses you practice by selecting sequences and poses from this book or similar books on the subject. Remember regularity is the key.

Part 3: Stabilizing the Pelvic Floor and Sacrum

One of the real challenges in the practice of yoga is to understand the need for stability and harmony between the pelvic floor, the sacroiliac joints, and the spine. I know from experience that about one-third of all yoga enthusiasts will find their hips and pelvic floor are out of balance in some way. And as the balance and tone of the pelvic floor, along with the stability of the SI joints, form the body's major weight transmitting structure between the earth and the spine, I have included this additional section.

The intent is to help you discriminate between back pain and sacroiliac joint pain, and introduce some sequences to address that particular imbalance. As always, read the entire section before beginning. If the descriptions in this section apply to you, ask a friend to help you complete the five muscle tests, and then begin with the Sacral Stabilization Sequence to see how you respond. As misperception is the most common function of mind according to yoga philosophy in the yoga sutra, please proceed slowly.

A sacral misalignment can be very squirrely, with the pain sometimes traveling side-to-side and/ or back to front. Therefore, along with practicing the sequences in the section, I suggest you consult with a yoga or other bodywork professional to help you find clarity and monitor your progress.

Part 4: The Bonus Section

Once you're familiar with the poses and the needs of your body, you can begin to add variety to your practice. There are two additional short sequences in this section that you can use to discover your body in new ways. Also, you'll find a chart guiding you in customizing your practice by choosing the best poses to create muscular balance for your particular needs.

Part 5: The Pose Sheets

I just love the KISS principle—keep it simple sweetie! Here you'll find all the sequences with only the photos of the poses for quick reference when practicing; you can also make copies of your favorites to take with you on a trip. The sequences are separated into short 15–25 minutes, and long 40–50 minutes. There are six short sequences in this section that you can choose from when your practice time is limited.

Yoga is intended to help us live a better, more integrated life and gain wisdom along the way. It takes into account the whole person, so even though our practice may not be perfect, the blessing of yoga will appear. The important message is to practice, practice, practice.

Self-Applied Back Care

As when we begin any journey, it's wise to have a map and understand the terrain. The principles that follow will offer you some points of understanding on how the body functions as a dynamic system.

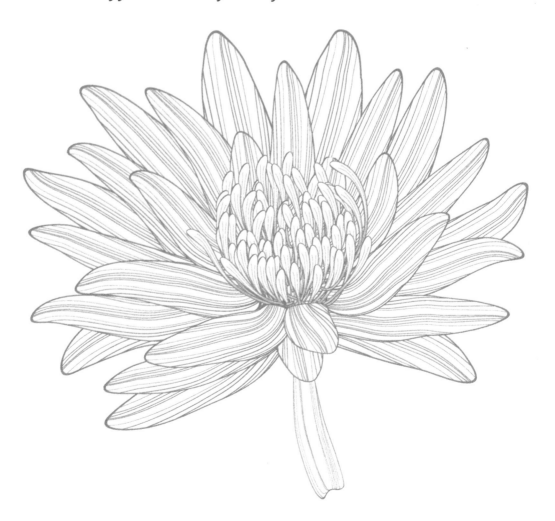

A Balanced System of Guide Wires

For all functional purposes, assume that the spine starts at the pelvic floor and ends at the atlas, upon which the cranium sits. Considering that whole range, it's never just the low back that is out of balance—everything else is affected as well. Picture an old-fashioned radio tower with the big guide wires staked into the ground. In order for the tower to be erect, the guide wires had to be balanced. One wire would have to have the same amount of tension as the other, so that the tower would stay straight up.

This is a clue about what happens with our spine in relation to gravity. If the main postural muscles are out of balance—the guide wires are off—it creates compression and wear and tear on our spines. Therefore, a person needs to have, not only abdominal strength (which is the conventional wisdom), but also a balance of tone and flexibility in the spinal and lateral muscles, along with mobility in the hips, in order to become upright and pain-free.

Two Phases of Back Pain

Most people experience back trouble in two distinct phases:

1. Back pain
2. A weak, painless back that is more susceptible to re-injury

When you injure yourself, the body part you've injured usually swells up. This swelling stops the joint or joints from moving. Your body is smart—it protects you. However, you do have to pay attention, because your body is trying to tell you something, and the way it does that is through pain. So, you clear your schedule, apply ice and then heat, consult with a professional, and rest.

Over some duration of time, the pain goes away, the muscle spasms relax, and you're back on your feet, but you end up with weak muscles. Then you have another incident. This time, it's a little worse than before. You rest for a while, the pain goes away again, and the muscles are weaker still. It progresses that way until people end up in a chronic pain pattern.

The good news is that you can change the pattern with your yoga practice. My students have often reported that through their consistent back care practices, not only did their pain diminish, but when they did experience another incident, their recovery time was much faster: maybe three days, for example, instead of three weeks.

The following chart comes directly from the National Safety Council's Back Power Program, and it shows the progression from the first incident of back pain to the chronic-pain state.

The Progression of Low Back Pain

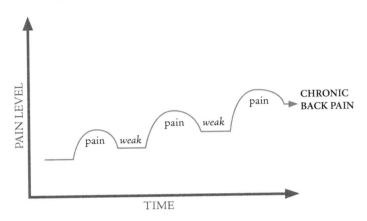

Reprinted with permission; Back Power Program.

Muscles in Spasm Remain in Spasm

The following problems characterize spastic muscles:

➤ They compromise the muscular balance and increase joint wear and tear.
➤ When they relax, the muscle is weak.
➤ Their length tends to remain short. The muscle forgets how to lengthen until acted upon by an outside force.

You have heard this story before: "All I did was bend over to pick up that paper clip, and there I was with a back spasm." The size and force of the spasm may be greater according to the weight of the object being lifted. However, regardless of the severity, a muscle that goes into spasm will often get locked into the spastic pattern. It simply forgets how to relax. It's not something we do in our mind—it's something that happens automatically.

The muscles remain short and contracted, even when the pain of the spasm is gone. That is how they stay until acted upon by another force, such as your yoga practice. In order for your spine to get healthy, balance has to be restored. If we allow the muscles to remain short and out of balance, we leave ourselves open for increased joint wear and tear, which leads to more chronic back conditions.

Scar Tissue Limits Mobility

Scar tissue is what your body puts in place to heal injuries, incisions, and the like. It has a chaotic cellular structure, which when fully formed, can seriously limit mobility. As fast as the body can lay it down given the specific circumstances, it will. It's trying to stabilize and mend torn connective tissue by creating an internal bandage.

Scar tissue is still forming and relatively pliable for six to eight months, possibly even up to one year, but the sooner you start moving the affected area, the better. That's why surgeons nowadays have patients get up and walk around as soon as possible after back surgery. Doctors have come to know that the body has its own wisdom, and if you get up and move, the body will start to recalibrate and maintain some range of motion as the scar tissue forms. In many cases, our bodies actually heal better through movement.

So, whether your scar tissue is from an injury or surgery, while it's still soft and pliable, start a simple yoga practice. When you do your yoga practice using alignment principles, you can safely extend, create length and space, and help maintain a healthy range of motion by guiding the scar tissue to a higher level of organization. This will allow for more movement in the future. Scar tissue is just another connective tissue that can be influenced and reorganized, especially when it's forming.

Once scar tissue is set, however, it becomes rigid, and when you stretch it, you'll experience more pain than when you stretch muscles, because it's stronger and creates more resistance. To create any change in established scar tissue takes a commitment of time and effort. The recommendation is to hold poses for long durations of time (2–10 minutes) to release the scar tissue without damaging the soft tissue around it.

The moral of the story is, when you've sustained an injury, after you've rested for one to three weeks, that's enough! Get on the mat. Find out what you can do that doesn't aggravate the injured area. Also, the older we get, the more rigid the scar tissue becomes. So, if you don't deal with it early on, it will just get worse. There is a good recommendation in a book I like to use in my teacher trainings: *The Runner's Yoga Book: A Balanced Approach to Fitness.* The authors recommend laying off your activities for up to three weeks, and then adding back a few stretches you can do that do not directly affect the injured area. They suggest you pay attention to how your injury is feeling, and add one pose every couple of days.

One of my students told me her doctor was amazed by her range of motion and excellent scores on her reflex and sensory tests, given her condition of several herniated discs from a car accident. She had continued to stretch after her accident, avoiding a buildup of scar tissue. She had a micro discectomy operation coming up, and he instructed her to return to yoga and qi gong, and whatever she'd been doing after two weeks of post-surgery recovery, because it was clear to him that whatever she'd been doing was working. Her case speaks to the idea that if you keep the body moving in an intelligent way, you can maintain a level of health, even in crisis. That student likely came out of her surgery so much better off than the average patient. When you have that connection with your body, you're friends with it, you know what the next right movement is, then you're ahead of the game by a mile. A yoga practice can be very empowering.

Breathe & Stretch to Relieve Pain & Stress

Yoga postures, called *asanas*, and full torso breathing, called *pranayama*, serve as useful tools for stress reduction. Yoga stretches are distinct from fitness stretches because they are practiced with an inner mental focus, which helps to create a shift toward the relaxation response and the parasympathetic nervous system. The physical emphasis is on balancing movement, while simultaneously elongating and strengthening the muscles and connective tissue using the breath. Yoga practice does not eliminate the stress in life, but it can shift our perception from feeling uncomfortable and threatened to an immediate and noticeable feeling of safety and calm.

The common denominator of all inducers of the relaxation response is an internal focus. Every time the mind wanders (and it will), bring your attention gently back to the focus point (on the breath). Directing attention internally is the physiological opposite of directing attention to the outside world looking for danger. When attention is directed inward, your body receives messages that you are safe and secure and that it is appropriate to relax. So muscles relax, blood pressure drops, nerves are calmed, anxiety is decreased, immunity is heightened and healing is enhanced.

~Mary Pullig Schatz, M.D., *Back Care Basics*

A well-defined set of physiological responses is elicited when our minds perceive a threat. The response from the sympathetic nervous system prepares us for fight or flight in order to cope with danger and protect ourselves. However, a chronically stressed state interferes with *homeostasis*, the body's ability to create internal stability and equilibrium, with resulting increased muscle tension. Postural strain also increases muscle tension, which is not evenly distributed, but will accumulate in vulnerable areas already weakened by present or past injuries. Sustained muscular tension tends to squeeze the blood vessels, reducing circulation and producing lactic acid buildup, which further increases the pain response, thereby reducing cellular regeneration.

In the stress cycle, parts of the brain, including the cerebral cortex, the hypothalamus, the pituitary gland, and the adrenal glands, go on alert. The brain signals the muscles to tighten and be ready to strike back. The blood vessels of the skin constrict, which leads to increased heart rate and more blood being pumped. This dramatically alters blood chemistry, affecting oxygen and carbon dioxide levels, blood volume, and pH. In an effort to cope with either a real or an imagined threat from the outside world, breathing becomes shallow. Unfortunately, this vicious cycle tends to become habitual and occurs unconsciously. The more pain we feel, the more stress is perceived.

Therefore, the starting point for reversing the stress cycle is to first alter the stressed breathing pattern. Relaxed, conscious breathing works by decreasing the respiration rate and increasing oxygenation while stretching the lungs and surrounding chest muscles. Add that to the balanced actions of yoga postures, which help to restore body-wide circulation and assist in the removal of toxins, which have built up in the static stress state. The biofeedback of relief increases a sense of self-empowerment. A shift from externally directed thought to self-directed creative thought brings the mind on board to effect an inner and outer transformation. In yoga, the relaxed body and mind link together, cells refuel, and nourishment is received, allowing us to lead inspired lives.

Physical Factors to Consider

Curves of the Spine

There are four spinal curves: *sacral, lumbar, thoracic,* and *cervical.* Each vertebral shape is unique to its location in the curve. The sacral curve, ending with the tailbone, curves out; the lumbar section curves in; the thoracic spine, where the ribs attach, curves out; and the cervical spine curves in. Therefore, when we deviate too far from the normal curves of the spine through either postural or functional stresses, we increase the risk of back pain.

Everyone enjoys the pleasure of standing up straight. It's a sign that all is well and we have the confidence to face life with equanimity. However, our bodies are structurally designed to be on all fours. So even though we stand upright, we still bear some quadruped physiology. For example, if

you were on all fours, then when you lifted your head, you would naturally create the cervical curve, gravity would create your lumbar curve, your spine would be suspended, and there would be no pressure on your sacrum.

Also, if you look at your muscle structure, you'll discover that the most powerful muscles are the pectoralis muscles in the chest, which draw the arms in toward the center line, and the adductors on the inside of the legs, the ones that keep the legs pulled in and connected to the body's midline. In contrast, the muscles on the outside of the arms and legs are much smaller and less powerful. To move into an upright position, we need to extend the more powerful muscles and cultivate healthy tone and action in the smaller muscles to establish structural balance and good posture in relationship to gravity. As we practice the yoga poses in this book, our focus will be to practice in a way that preserves and balances the curves of our spine. Read more on muscles and how they affect posture on pages 10 and 11.

The Problem with Gravity

Being upright in the field of gravity is a challenge every day. When we're young, it's easy. And then 30 years go by—40 years, 50 years—and gravity has been pulling in the other direction for all that time. People who don't stretch tend to shrink as they get older. Gravity has been pulling down; the spine has been compressed, over and over. In order to be effortlessly upright in the field of gravity, we have to learn to extend our spines in a balanced way.

The prolonged effects of gravity, along with muscular imbalances and load bearing stresses, cause the discs to become thinner, bone spurs begin to develop, and the facet joints along the spine that articulate each vertebra to the one below it begin to pinch. In fact, with 80 percent of the nerve endings along the spine located in the facet joints, this pinching due to contracted muscles along the spine as a result of poor posture and gravity contributes to the majority of non-clinical back pain.

Sitting

Sitting causes people to lose more length in their spine than does any other single activity. Everyone does a lot of sitting—in a car, at the computer, sewing, reading. Sitting always causes us to deviate from our normal back curves. So the lumbar and cervical curves are pushed in the opposite direction from nature's design, and the muscles in those areas weaken, making those parts of our spine most vulnerable to back pain. Additionally, prolonged sitting shortens the hip flexors and weakens our abdominal muscles, creating too much forward tilt in the pelvis when we stand, thus pinching the facet joints in the lumbar region, which also contributes to back pain. The door can swing both ways.

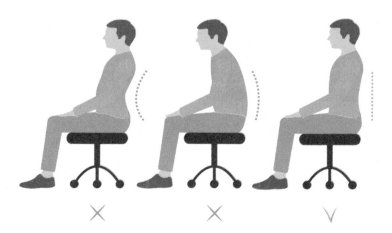

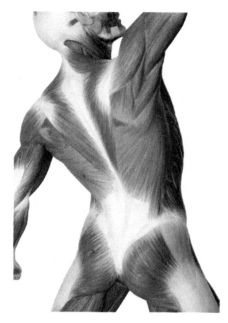

Fascia is a tough connective tissue that spreads throughout the body in a three-dimensional web. About 20 percent of the weight of the human body is fascia.

Know about Fascia

In this age of the Internet, we're all familiar with the amazing possibilities of connection. When we relate to our bodies as a web of fascia, or connective tissue, we can discover and understand connections that we never imagined existed.

Fascia is a tough connective tissue that spreads throughout the body in a three-dimensional web from head to foot without interruption. The fascia surrounds every muscle, bone, nerve, blood vessel, and organ of the body, all the way down to the cellular level. Therefore, malfunction of the fascial system due to trauma, posture, or inflammation can cause it to bind down, resulting in abnormal pressure on nerves, muscles, bones, or organs. This can lead to pain or malfunction throughout the body, sometimes with bizarre side effects and seemingly unrelated symptoms.

Note: None of the standard tests, such as x-rays, myelograms, CT scans, magnetic resonance imaging (MRI), or electromyography (EMG), show the fascial restrictions.

There is a lot of fascia in the body: About 20 percent of the weight of the human body is fascia and fibrous connective tissue. "A body-wide responsive physiological network on par in terms of importance and scope with the circulatory and nervous systems," according to Thomas Myers, author of *Anatomy Trains*. There are seven major fascial trains in the body that are vitally involved in all aspects of motion and act as shock absorbers—physically, physiologically, and psychologically. Along with the seven major facial trains that run from head to toe, both superficial and deep, there are also four major horizontal planes of fascia. These horizontal planes of organization in the body are known in yoga as the *four diaphragms*. Due to the conductive and connective nature of fascia, any pressure of expansion, namely stretching, along one segment of a fascial train will benefit the other segments of that train as well.

When we experience stress due to a physical or emotional event that is interrupted or unresolved, the fascia will begin to pleat, or fold back on itself, creating a bunching effect that reduces the flow of breath, fluids, and electrical information. Repetitive motion, muscular imbalances, age, and trauma also contract and pleat fascia. Once fascial adhesions form, then an injury becomes chronic.

The spinal cord or central nervous system is also surrounded by fascial tissue, called the *dura mater*, which attaches to the second sacral segment and the inside of the cranium. The dura mater has the protective strength of a tire and tends to remain mostly unharmed, with the exception of possible pleating from a fall or other injury. As we know, extreme dysfunction in spinal tissue caused by traumas, including surgery, can have widespread neurological effects and a resulting loss of function.

According to the research of Dr. Ida Rolf, a biochemist and the creator of a body-work technique called Rolfing, fascia is made up of liquid crystal, which is either fluid or solid, and it is also *piezoelectric*, which means electrons can jump from one cell to another throughout the fascial matrix. Fascia responds well to pressure, stretching, and twisting, which allow the tissues to be hydrated and transformed from "sol to gel" (solid to fluid), creating a flow of bio-energy throughout the mind-body complex. Otherwise the fascia remains bound down, causing pain and restriction.

Through my experience as a massage therapist, yoga practitioner, and yoga instructor, I have come to know that an extremely high percentage of people suffering from pain or lack of mobility have been experiencing fascial problems. A yoga practice acts on connective tissue as much as the muscles, which explains why so many students improve dramatically after attending only a handful of yoga classes.

Intent in the Practice of Yoga

Over the years, I have witnessed time and again how yoga, when taught and practiced in a systematic, balanced, and mindful way—can promote the body's ability to heal. The intentions we set at the beginning of our yoga practice inform our actions and the order of those actions. It is with such an intention that I have organized the poses and sequences in this book.

Below are three steps you can follow to start on the road to recovery from back pain.

1. First and foremost, create length and space.
2. Gradually increase range of motion.
3. Rebuild strength and stability.

Create Length and Space

As we understand how back pain progresses through muscular imbalance, fascial pleating, poor posture, and the subtle yet constant pull of gravity, we can understand the need to decompress our spines by creating length. When we create length we also create space.

Creating length and space allows the joints of the spine to decompress, which relieves nerve pain or pinching and reduces inflammation. Ever notice how good it feels to lie down on the floor and let your spine relax after a long day of sitting? This is because you are creating passive length in your spine.

In yoga we create length and space through positioning as well as by extending our arms and legs to extend our spine. It's like magic: when our legs are long and strong, our spines receive the support, and we stand taller. When our legs fold, our spine shrinks. Therefore, we can extend our spines indirectly by learning to extend our legs, as you will discover in some of the sequences offered in this book.

Increase Range of Motion

You can't do what you can't do, and you can't get anywhere without going step by step. When the muscles are tight, or if they're in spasm and are locked up—you can't force them to open. You need to cultivate the muscles, just like you would cultivate hard, dry, soil. Working little by little, use the pressure of the stretch against the resistance. Move in and out of the stretch with intentional breathing, to allow the fascia and muscles to begin to let go.

Your body is meant to be a fluid, living organism, but when parts of it become stuck, it's like they're spot-welded together. They need to be opened up, because that is what allows healing to happen. As we maintain a consistent practice with discipline and patience, the short muscles will begin to lengthen, and along with this lengthening, our range of movement will increase and our vulnerability will decrease.

Rebuild Strength and Stability

Once your pain level is down to a 1, 2, or 3—on a scale of 1 to 10—while you're practicing, your body is pretty happy, and you're ready to begin toning muscles again. Rebuilding strength is easy. In a matter of two or three days, we can almost double our muscle tone with dynamic weight-bearing yoga poses. Unlike stretching, which is a process of patient undoing, all toning requires is the willpower to press on. We're simply designed

to rebuild; our muscles like to contract—it's what they do best! We know that when the muscles are happy, it makes us feel good. When the body is happy, then we are happy.

It's my experience that creating length and space and getting the parts that are rigid to become pliable again is what requires the most effort. Stretching muscles, making their resting length longer, and creating relative muscular balance, does take time—three months or more—depending on your personal practice, stress levels, and chemistry.

Caution: Be mindful when you begin to add toning poses to your practice. Too much to soon could cause compression and reactivate the pain response. Add poses one at a time, and observe.

Back Pain Profile

As is typical for our species, we spend a fair amount of time doing what we can to avoid pain. However, pain finds us over and over again. All pain is not the same; there are different messages hidden in the sensation of pain, and therefore different ways to understand it.

When a person experiences back pain due to an impact or an overuse or misuse injury, the pain can linger sometimes for years. Often, people don't realize that their habitual movements or standard exercise programs are contributing to their back problems. No one wishes to harm him or herself, or experience back pain, but it happens.

Continued back pain typically leads to a fear of movement in an effort to avoid possible reinjury. Once this fear has established itself, then a person's pain profile becomes compounded with added muscular tension, emotional stress, reduced activity, an inability to work, and a loss of muscle tone and self-confidence.

I would say that one of my biggest roles as a yoga teacher when I offer back care classes is to help people recognize that they don't need to be fearful about moving. I give people permission to move. Sometimes they have been living for months with the pain and they are scared to move. If they knew how to move, if they knew what to move, and that they could do so safely, they would do it. Everyone wants to heal and be pain free.

To heal, we must understand and accept that our bodies are intelligent and are always speaking to us. My body is my friend: it has been with me since the beginning, and it has always done what I've asked of it. Think about it. If you have had a lot of back pain, just remember that your body is your friend. It's not

going to lie to you. If you overdo some movement, it's going to give you a signal. If you do the right thing, you're going to feel good. And if you don't feel better, you're not doing the right thing. It can be that simple. Look inward, feel, and listen for the physical sensations. They are your feedback.

Understanding Positive, Negative, and Post-Exercise Pain

In the beginning, all pain seems to be negative, yet some pain is positive—especially the pain of movement that leads us toward healing. On the following pages you'll find three definitions to help you recognize which type of pain you're having at any given moment and guide you on how to proceed.

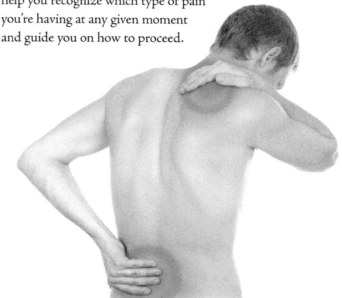

Positive Pain

Positive pain is a dull, aching feeling. When you stop stretching, the pain stops, and your body feels good. Over time, as the muscles lengthen, your overall pain will decrease. While you're stretching, it hurts. When you stop stretching, there is no pain, and you feel better. This is positive.

Even when you're doing a yoga pose and discover a pain level of a 6–7 (on the 1–10 scale), it could be positive. You are not creating the pain—you are discovering it. Pain is only an indicator of some part of your physical or mental/emotional body that is calling for attention and healing. When the pain you discover in your body has intensity, remember to play the edge by backing off to a place where you can breathe deeply. That could mean backing down to a level of 5–6 or 3–4: it's your choice. However, go slowly, stay with the stretch, breathe, keep listening within, and know that your body's healing forces are being mobilized, and the muscles and fascia that need to lengthen are doing so. New students often comment, "It feels so good when I stop!" Look for that experience.

Negative Pain

Negative pain is a sharp, electric feeling, typically close to the joint. It may jab, bite, or burn, or you may get a feeling of numbness when you stretch the area. You might refer to the location of your negative pain or injury as your "Signal Spot."

Negative pain is our ally, as it stops us in our tracks and prevents further injury. When we have some form of nerve impingement from a herniated disc, bone spurs, or a spinal misalignment, the pain can radiate along the nerve pathway as inflammation. *Sciatica* is one of the labels we give to radiating nerve pain that is inflamed. It's always best to wait until any inflammation has subsided before beginning or returning to a yoga practice.

As discussed earlier, sometimes the inflammation and pain subsides, yet the misalignment, herniation, or bone spurs that caused it are still present. When we begin our yoga stretching program, we need to proceed with caution and give particular attention to maintaining good alignment, and choose poses that avoid direct stress to the injured or compromised area.

You will know if you have stressed your injury, because when you come out of the pose, there will be a twinge or throb in your "Signal Spot". In the first two breaths

after coming out of the pose and returning to neutral, your body will tell you if it liked what you did or not. So proceed, but always go slowly and breathe deeply. Back off the stretch 10 percent, maybe even to a level of 2–3. Sometimes less is more.

Caution: Typically, backing off the stretch like that will allow you to progress without any more negative pain. If it doesn't help, and you still have negative pain when you come out of the pose, stop doing the pose until you can consult with your yoga teacher or health professional.

Post-Exercise Pain

Post-exercise pain is usually considered positive pain when a general ache or soreness in the muscles appears within two to three days of new physical activity. There may be a doubt in your mind whether the pain is okay, but if you really listen to your body and look within, you'll find that the nerves are not inflamed and there is no radiating pain.

When starting a yoga stretching routine to assist with healing, it's likely you will experience some soreness in your muscles, depending on their level of previous conditioning. Soreness is an indicator that the circulation and muscle tone need to improve, and it should encourage you to practice more regularly. In those cases where soreness lasts more than four or five days, you likely overextended yourself with too aggressive a practice, lost your alignment and the length and space in your spine, causing nerve irritation, or you have stressed a muscle that was already long and weak. You may also need to consider other lifestyle factors along with mental/emotional stress. Please refer to the section on Addressing Pain with Your Mind on the next page.

Pain Receptors Don't Discriminate

Often, when a weak muscle is exercised, the pain receptors will fire and send signals to the brain, mimicking the same response as an injury. The brain must then discriminate. Use your breath and inward focus to find your way.

Negative pain is easy to recognize once you learn to listen, but have you ever noticed that pain receptors don't really discriminate between positive and negative pain? The first time you stretch a tight muscle, it just hurts. You only come to know the pain as positive when the stretch has ended, the pain stops, and you feel better. Our minds must learn to differentiate.

When we have sore muscles after a new exercise, we typically think nothing of it. But when the exercise makes us sore near or around our "Signal Spot," we naturally get worried. You think, "Why am I sore? That's where I hurt my back. Oh, surely this can't be good." The first thing the mind does is judge, especially when the fear of re-injury is present: "I'm feeling something, and it's not comfortable. Surely it's bad." This is how the mind gets in the way of healing. You have to remember to stop and investigate, "What really, is the exact sensation?" And, "If I move my low back a little bit, I can feel those muscles are sore, but I don't feel that twinge or any radiating pain down my leg, so maybe it's okay." You have to do that with your mind—this is where self-discipline and self-study comes in. Continue your practice and investigate the responses of both your mind and your body.

The pain receptors are the same, regardless of whether we're experiencing the pain of an injury or the pain of healing. If healing were not painful, then there would be no pain medications. If you have ever had a surgery, you hope the doctor gives you pain medicine. Why? Because, as your body is knitting, producing new cells or scar tissue, the pain of healing is often more intense than the pain of the injury. The longer you can go without pain medicine, and listen to your body and let it be your guide, the faster you will heal. The less you mask it over, the more your body will tell you what it needs, what is working and what isn't. Of course, be reasonable—use common sense, but know that the pain you have is an indicator and a guide.

Weak Muscles Complain—No Fear

When you begin to rebuild strength in a weak muscle, it will complain, often by cramping. This is temporary.

Again, people naturally become fearful: "Is this okay? Am I going to hurt myself?" I have a rule of thumb about that: When you start rebuilding strength—say you're starting to build some strength in the buttocks and the lower back muscles—my rule of thumb is to go slow. Hold the new poses for short durations, usually 10 seconds at a time, and then repeat the same pose three days in a row. At the end of the third day, the muscles will be less sore and have more strength. If, by the end of the third day, you're starting to get nerve pain and inflammation, then it's too much too soon. Back off. Stop. Regroup. Go back to simply creating length and space in your muscles and joints. Try again another time or in another way to gradually build strength; consult with your yoga teacher or health care provider.

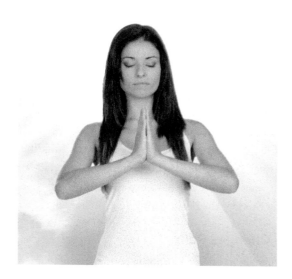

Addressing Pain with Your Mind

When you begin to experience any intensity of pain in a yoga pose and fear begins to arise, there is a simple four-step formula to follow.

1. Stop and breathe.
2. Don't resist the resistance.
3. Suspend judgment.
4. Wait and feel for a release. It will come.

Stop and breathe: Stop the range of motion before any negative pain is triggered, but hold the pose right there at the edge of the resistance. Inhale and bring your mind to your breath and your breath to your body. **Calm yourself.**

Don't resist: In your mind say, "I am not going to resist. I'm not going to hold my breath or grip my stomach. I'm not going to tighten my throat or clench my teeth." Catch yourself in all those ways your body wants to tense up and resist when we try to force our way through something. Repeat, "I am not going to resist, I am going to breathe." Learn to let go of the resistance. It is both physical and mental. Back off 10 percent as needed and bring your body to your breath—**feel.**

Suspend judgment: In our culture, we hold very high standards and tend to be overly critical toward ourselves. We're also conditioned to avoid discomfort. When we find ourselves in pain, we may think we have failed or that our body has failed us. I have not found this to be true. My body always works on my behalf, keeping up with me as best it can. Your body is not broken. Compromised maybe, yet it's very capable of healing and moving to a new level of function.

Suspend judgment, be patient, and just breathe. Instead of judging, ask: "I wonder what message my body has for me?" Then, not only are you suspending judgment, but now you're looking to **your inner self** for guidance. You're understanding that it's possible to receive guidance from your own true self, and that it's possible for you to evolve and change. This is the definition of a spiritual practice.

Wait for the release: This one is very important. **Wait for the release.** Go in and arrive at the place where you think the negative pain might start. Stop. Breathe deeply. Suspend judgment. And then wait. Just wait. I guarantee something will change. Give your body time for the healing force to mobilize, and it will.

Breath Changes Pain

When you're in a yoga pose, finding your alignment and creating extension, you'll meet your wall of resistance. This is the point where you're experiencing a sensation of discomfort ranging between 4–7 on the pain scale, before any negative pain begins.

Pause here. Begin by backing out of the stretch 10 percent so you can breathe easily. Knock on the door of the tight places in your body, bring your mind to your breath and your breath to your body, and follow the four steps listed above for addressing pain.

To reduce the tension you feel in your muscles, take slow, deep breaths, making your exhales longer than your inhales. In this way, you'll access the relaxation response, and discover that the muscles will begin to let go and your discomfort will settle down. Breath gives softness and release to the body, especially when we exhale.

If the tension in the muscle is being stubborn, try breathing in and out with a pause. Add a brief and intentional pause at the top of the inhale. (In yoga, this pause is called *anatarah kumbaka*.) In that small pause, just imagine that your breath popped into your whole body. So, it's not just in your lungs anymore; it's all the way out to the edges of your skin. How does that make you feel? Hopefully, more relaxed and present. Slowly exhale. You can also pause at the end of the exhalation (*bahya kumbaka*) to deeply calm yourself and release all resistance.

Three Ways to Approach Stretching

Contrary to popular opinion, there is more to stretching than simply extending your leg out and bending over. Understanding how muscles stretch will help you choose right action in your yoga poses to create release and relief. Let's examine the function of *reciprocal inhibition, adaptation,* and *contract-relax PNF stretching.*

1. Reciprocal Inhibition

Reciprocal inhibition is the primary physiological principle that will help you choose the right exercise for the right situation. When one group of muscles is contracted, the opposite muscles lengthen. It happens automatically, no thought is required. Furthermore, when an overly tight muscle is stretched, its opposing muscle is toned. The door swings both ways. I've included a few examples below to illustrate.

Note: *The take-away message is that we can contract one muscle group to easily and effortlessly relieve tension or spasm in its opposite group. It works every time. So if you find yourself in a situation where muscles are cramping and complaining, look for a yoga pose that contracts the opposite muscles and you'll find some relief.*

Tight Hamstrings: When the hamstrings are really short, the quads tend to be very soft and weak. New yoga students often struggle to firm their quads when bending forward to stretch their hamstrings. They lift their kneecaps to firm their quads, which then fall almost immediately. They get it and lose it over and over again. They can't sustain it, because the hamstring muscle is so short that it's preventing the quadriceps from contracting and maintaining its tone.

What does that tell you? First, because these students are not contracting their quadriceps—even though their feeling a great deal of sensation in their hamstrings—the hamstrings are actually gripping and shortening to protect the backs of the knees. So, unless and until the quadriceps and the kneecaps are lifted and engaged, the hamstrings won't release and lengthen. Some students I've taught have been doing yoga for 20 years and their hamstrings are still short. They keep doing forward bends, but the hamstrings still haven't lengthened very much, because they never knew that they had to contract the opposite muscles in order to get the hamstrings to let go.

One standard pose that stretches the hamstrings is Strap Work 1, Supta Padangusthasana (see page 24). To do this pose, the quad muscles will eventually need to contract. New students often experience so much sensation in their hamstrings that they allow the leg to simply hang in the hip and knee joints. Again, the door swings both ways, so when you fully extend the back of the leg, the quadriceps will begin to tone, tapping the reflex arc of reciprocal inhibition, thus causing the hamstring muscles to truly lengthen.

Neck Tension: When a person suffers from excess tension in the back of the neck from years of poor posture, often presenting as forward head carriage, lying down and lifting the head to look at the feet (see page 29) brings relief. By contracting the front of the neck and loading the muscles with the weight of the head, the person is able to release and lengthen the muscles in the back of the neck. Often, a student experiences the sensation of the muscles lengthening as discomfort or pain. Again, the mind must discriminate to see if the discomfort ends when the pose ends, thus identifying the pain as positive.

Overstretched Muscles: Sometimes a muscle goes into pain or spasm because it has been weakened by too much stretching. An example would be the pain we get in the back of the neck from long hours spent looking down. Those muscles have been overloaded and lengthened by holding the weight of the head. When the back of the neck is fatigued or aching in this manner, a baby fish pose (page 29) can be applied to help tone those muscles and relieve the pain. Contracting those muscles returns them to a healthy resting length, also releasing any tension in the front of the neck, and the pain signals will stop.

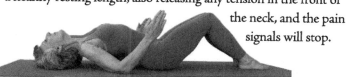

Tight Chest Muscles: If you spend a lot of your time hunched over or looking down, the chest muscles and those in the front of the neck will contract and become tight. Fish pose can also help open those muscles through reciprocal inhibition. In this example, I ask my students to use the leverage of their elbows and the back of their head to tone the posterior muscles of the neck and shoulder blades, thereby retraining the seventh cervical vertebra to move inward, for more healthy function. When we tone the mid-trapezius, rhomboid, and levator scapulae muscles in the back, we're also releasing tight scalene and pectoralis muscles in the front.

Low Back Spasms: You can easily and naturally release tension in the low back muscles by performing abdominal toning exercises such as yogi curl ups, Ardha Navasana (half boat pose), and alternate leg lifts (refer to the Abdominal Progressions on page 33). These poses help to create abdominal support for the low back, and release spasms and fatigue in those compromised back muscles.

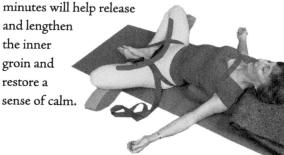

2. Adaptation

Adaptation is the practice of holding poses and watching your breath until the muscles let go and the discomfort subsides. Holding poses for longer durations (2–15 minutes, or longer) is helpful when scar tissue is involved, or as part of a restorative practice to reduce the stress response. For example, holding Supported Supta Baddha Konasana (see page 47) for 5–10 minutes will help release and lengthen the inner groin and restore a sense of calm.

3. Contract-Relax PNF Stretching

The full name of this approach is *Contract-Relax Approach to Proprioceptive Neuromuscular Facilitation*. This describes an action where we deliberately contract a muscle while stretching, and then let go of it slowly, creating a longer resting length of the muscle. Although this method is mentioned here, it remains secondary to the poses and actions we'll explore in this book for back pain relief.

In the practice of yoga, the proper understanding of anatomical alignment and principles enables students to be successful in their personal practice and develop their skills of observation. Understanding alignment also provides students and yoga practitioners with a map for discovering and unwinding constricted areas of their own bodies.

Our bones and muscles are more or less symmetrical, meaning each muscle has a matching one on the other side of the body. When we perform our poses systematically, we're able to discover where we're strong and where we're weak. When we successfully apply the alignment principles, we begin to create for ourselves harmony and balance, avoiding the pitfalls and difficulties associated with over-stretching or under-stretching.

Applying the alignment principles helps us create length and space safely, making it easier to identify our strong and weak areas and respond accordingly. The fascia and muscles realign following our requests for action and extension, and our bodies then reorganize to a higher level. We end up with a deeper organization and integration of our structure and create change in our patterns of movement and posture. So as you create more and more balance, more organization, your pain will diminish and your ability to move will increase.

A Collection of Tubes

To simplify the alignment principles, we can relate to the body as a system of "tubes." Imagine your body as a collection of large and small tubes. Consider your torso to be a large, squeezable water tube. The volume remains the same, but the shape can change dramatically. When practicing yoga, maintain an image in your mind of this tube to help you perceive areas of collapse or overexpansion. When observing a limb, think of it as having four sides and a center. Do your best to align around the center of each limb and the center of your torso.

The same desired action applies to the small tubes of the body—the blood vessels and nerves. When a small tube is collapsed, there can be either referred nerve pain, like a pinched nerve, or the blockage of circulation. A pinch is an alignment problem. When or if you feel a pinch in a joint, it's not your body's fault: it means your alignment is off. You have four directions to move in to discover how to "unpinch" the tube, i.e., to open the front, back, inside, or outside of the joint or body part in question.

Reflect upon and adjust your alignment to open the tubes, relieve pinching, and enhance a good flow of *prana*, or energy.

The Clock Face

Core strength and pelvic stability represent a key component of back health, aided by proper alignment. To help you balance your hips and lumbar spine, picture an image of a large clock face on the front of your pelvis: the navel is 12:00, the pubic bone is 6:00, and the hip bones are 3:00 and 9:00. The desired alignment action is to flatten the front of the clock face so that it remains perpendicular or parallel to the floor. To draw the center of your clock face in and up, learn to lift the soft tissue, i.e., the bottom of your belly and pelvic floor. Using the muscles and organs of your base will help to stabilize your low back and help support your spine. When low back pain is present, keep the hips level in all poses so both sides of the spine extend evenly, in other words, keep 3:00 and 9:00 on the same horizontal line.

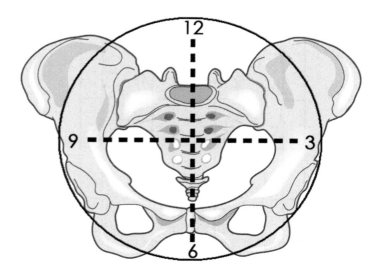

The Vertical Lines

In order to maintain or create good posture, it's important to develop awareness and alignment of the vertical lines in your body. You can practice this basic alignment principle right now by finding your plum line.

Stand in front of a floor-length mirror and view your body from the side. Place your ankles, knees, hips, pelvic floor, center of the shoulders, and ears all in one vertical line. Bring your clock face perpendicular to the floor and lift up your entire skeleton to find optimal extension to create length and space in your spine.

Now, view your body from the front, and imagine the centers of both legs as parallel lines running from the ankle through the center of the hip, to the nipple region, and up alongside your neck and head, like railroad tracks. In practice, if a leg twists or crosses the midline of the body, the clock face will be thrown off and the spine will receive the torque or compression. I call this a train wreck. Therefore, when aligning or activating the muscles of a limb, think of them as independent tubes that relate to each other and to the central tube. When performing poses, examine the inner and outer, front and back, and central lines of your limbs, and do your best to balance around the central line. Look at your body in the mirror both ways to help you determine what you need to adjust to be in balance, and bring that awareness into your practice.

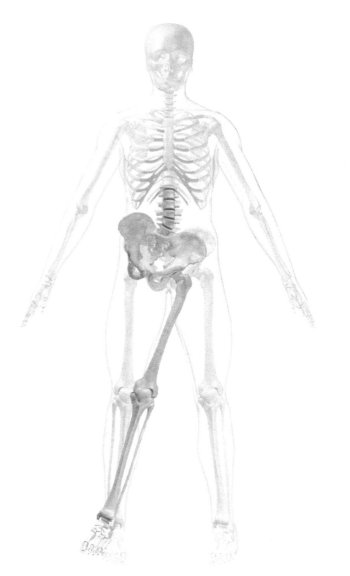

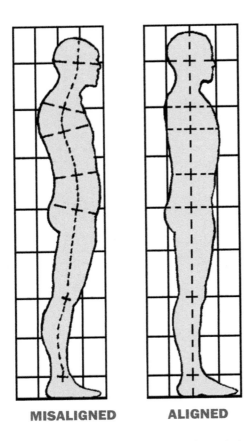

MISALIGNED   **ALIGNED**

To balance our bodies, it's important to observe both the vertical and horizontal lines and their relationships.

The Horizontal Lines

The four diaphragms that establish the horizontal structure of the central tube are the final component of anatomical alignment presented here. The first diaphragm, the *pelvic floor*, sets the foundation for the spine and determines the position of the upper three diaphragms. The muscles of the pelvic floor and pelvic ring form the weight transfer station of the human body and stabilize our body when we stand, sit, and walk. The relationship between the clock face and the pelvic floor give support and length to the lower back and spine.

The second diaphragm is the *respiratory diaphragm*, a powerful muscle that circularly expands the ribs, massages the internal organs, and responds to both voluntary and involuntary controls. In stressful situations, when our sympathetic nervous system is firing, the fibers of the respiratory diaphragm contract. Because this diaphragm attaches to all five lumbar vertebrae, excess contraction from sustained stress or a stressful event can create discomfort in our mid and lower backs.

The third diaphragm of the throat surrounding the thoracic outlet, describes an area of the body, rather than a muscle or membrane. This diaphragm is formed by the relationship between the collarbones, the spinous process of the shoulder blades, and the point of the outer tip of the shoulder. When this area lies parallel to the floor and centered over the other two diaphragms, the tubes of the neck remain elongated and neutral, which allows nerve impulses and prana to flow unimpeded into our head and arms.

The fourth diaphragm, a membrane called the *tentorium*, forms an arching bridge that supports the underside of the brain. Tension in the respiratory diaphragm translates into tension in the tentorium, as in a stress headache.

An awareness of the four diaphragms offers a three-dimensional reference to help us align the central tube of the body, allowing us to modify how we stand or sit to minimize discomfort in our spine.

The Subtle Actions

In yoga, the skin is considered the fifth organ of perception. Every inch of our skin is intelligent. My guru, B.K.S. Iyengar, considered the pores of the skin to be like eyes, capable of "seeing" in many directions. A common error students make when they first practice yoga is to simply hang in their joints, rather than extend their limbs and activate their skin. Here are seven subtle actions that will fully activate your skin and fascia, increasing the effectiveness of your practice, as well as reduce the discomfort of a positive stretch.

1. The legs extend the spine. In any yoga pose, do your best to extend the legs completely, as if you were reaching for infinity. *The extension of the legs is critical to the extension of the spine.*

2. The feet control the hips. Spreading and extending the soles of your feet, along with lifting the inner and outer arches, provide neuromuscular access to the muscles of the hips, helping to guide the alignment of the legs and the release of energy for the spine. *Wake up your feet in asana.*

3. Bring the thighbone to rest in the center of the hip socket. Think about standing: if the leg turns in too far, the back thigh misaligns and the low back tightens. If the leg turns out too far, the front thigh misaligns, the inner groins protrude forward, and the spine collapses. Both extremes disturb the "railroad tracks" and lead to instability in the hips and pelvic floor, with a correlating loss of alignment and support for the spine. *Bring your inner groins to the center of the pelvic floor so your thighs are directly under your hips.*

4. The knees align the legs. Position your knees so they point straight ahead. When standing, take the pressure off your back knee by micro bending slightly so the top shinbone moves forward to bring your front shin perpendicular to the floor. The top thighbone moves back as mentioned above. *Align the shin and thigh so the central tube of the leg remains straight.*

5. The arms expand the chest. Just as we extend the legs to extend our spine, expanding the arms out from the shoulders will release and expand the chest, supporting the expression of heart. *Open the chest and shoulders by expanding the arms.*

6. The hands activate the shoulders. Evenly extend all four sides of your wrist and elbow, joining the fingers together when possible to further soften and release the muscles of the neck and shoulders. *Balance the extension of your wrists and elbows to release the shoulders.*

7. The shoulder blades live on the back body. Remember how we were designed to be on all fours? When we stand upright, our shoulder blades need to draw back and down so our front chest can remain open, thus stabilizing the shoulder joint by maintaining good posture. *Pin the inner edge of the shoulder blade to the back ribs to maintain the stability of the chest and shoulder.*

When we bring our mind to our breath and our breath to our body, we bring consciousness to our skin. The sensations we feel in our skin tell us of our position in space. If our skin is very tight the indication is that we are over stretching and "bulging out" in that area. Conversely, if one area is tight,

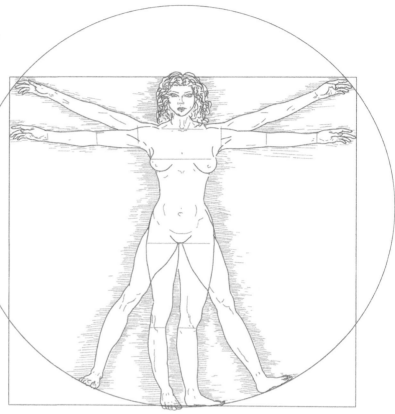

another area is collapsing. By listening to those sensations we can find our way to more balance in alignment and action.

In yoga, good alignment allows the prana or life energy to flow both vertically and horizontally, balancing the movement toward individuation (the vertical lines) with the sense of inclusion and compassion (the horizontal lines). Together they create the openness and expanse of the body-mind so we connect to the greater field of who we are.

Understanding Your Type

In the practice of yoga, three things appear to be true: You can overdo an action, underdo the same action, or be uncertain of which action to take. To help you understand the needs of your own body in healing back pain, let's consider three contrasting profiles.

The Ultra-Contracted

This group comprises, among others, 80 percent of the men who come to yoga because they have blown out their back.

There are always exceptions, but in general, men tend to be very stable and strong in the pelvis, hips, hamstrings, and quads, and oftentimes are muscle-bound. The lack of flexibility can force compensatory movement in the spine, the more movable area. So, they absorb all movement in their lumbar spine, causing extreme compression of the discs, leading to herniations.

For ultra-contracted individuals, the challenge is to not push, but rather breathe and go slow. Yoga is meant to ease and lengthen overly contracted muscles in the hips and legs so a person can bend from somewhere other than the low back. But, this lengthening can't occur unless we can slow down and be present in the practice.

Loosey-Goosey

This describes a large number of women who may be doing too much "stretchy" yoga without stabilizing, or who may be naturally prone to hyperextension and are particularly unstable in the pelvis. Many are past menopause, which causes muscle tone to diminish—we lose what we don't use more quickly after menopause. Those looser muscles and ligaments allow the joints to move too much and slip around, which causes pressure on the small tubes in unfavorable ways, and ultimately, leads to pain.

It's often difficult for the loosey-goosey yoga type to accept that, until their yoga practice and healing journey establishes stability in their pelvis, lifting, even as little as 20 pounds, may not be a good idea.

The Combo Pack

This is the person who has some areas or muscles that are tight and some that are too loose. When we consider structure and function, muscles that are overly short or contracted limit movement in that particular direction, which causes excessive movement in the opposite direction where there is less resistance. When the body produces a pain signal, it might be in either location for different reasons. If the pain is in the long muscles, it shows signs of distress because those muscles are over working trying to create stability. If the pain is in the short muscles, it indicates an overly strong muscle that needs to gradually stretch and release.

The guidance for healing is always to identify the short muscles to give them length, and the loose muscles to give them strength or tone. The relative balance created yields functional ability and reduced incidences of back pain.

Yoga Full Circle

So, we go from observing the structure of the body, to how our mind relates, to how we can use our breath; and that leads us to the inner self, to our own evolution as a person—to healing as an integral part of our spiritual practice.

Creating length and space? Un-spot-welding the body? This is not easy, and you have to pay attention and practice yoga with your mind as well as your body. You have to bring your mind into the present, you have to listen to your body, listen within, and practice compassion and kindness. If you push too hard in yoga, you'll hurt something, just like any other activity. Extend compassion to yourself as you look at your life: "Why do I keep creating the same tension over and over and over again? What are the seed thoughts that I'm feeding that continue to manifest as discomfort and tension in my body?" This could be the beginning of a rich journey.

Every injury can be a gift. Many people who have had life-threatening illnesses say it's the best thing that ever happened to them. They go within and find their true center, their true source, and they awaken. They awaken to their life in a gracious and positive way. That potential is there for all of us.

As part of your healing journey with back pain, focus your mind, listen inside, watch your thoughts and their effects, and visualize and rehearse the healing result you desire. Enjoy the feelings of freedom that will arise mentally and physically. Accept what you can't change and discover all the hidden possibilities of what you can change. Patanjali's *Yoga Sutra 1.14* offers guidance toward this end: "Consistent uninterrupted practice over time brings the goal of yoga close at hand."

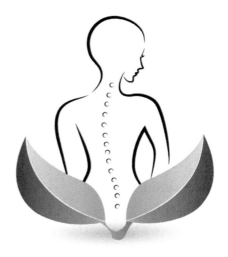

part 1, the poses
Self-Applied Back Care

In this section we explain the fundamentals of low back anatomy to help you understand how your posture and alignment impact your back. We explore how yoga improves back health and we offer four yoga sequences you can start practicing today to deal with back pain and begin to heal. In addition, we introduce practices and poses to promote deep relaxation, de-stress with ease, and expand your breathing capacity.

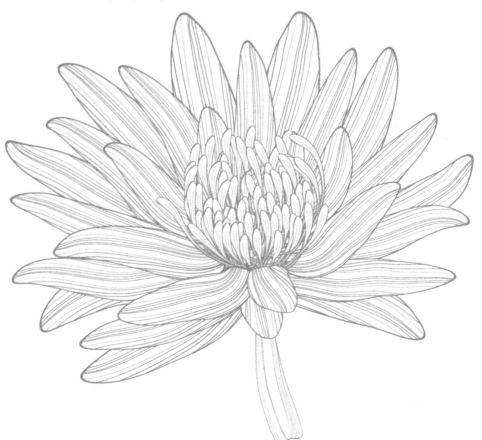

Anatomy & Key Muscles Affecting the Low Back

Understanding which muscles are responsible for various postural deviations offer guidance to help you identify, along with your practice, the short or long muscles in your own body. This knowledge will help you choose the best yoga poses to counterbalance / balance them for optimal function. I've listed the muscle groups in the order of importance to someone suffering from back pain.

Hamstring Group

The *hamstring* group is a band of three strong muscles that runs from the sitz bones (*ischial tuberosities*) to insert on the medial and lateral bones of the lower leg.

➢ **Short** hamstrings pull down on the sitz bones, causing the lumbar portion of the spine to over flex when bending forward, which weakens the lower back, often resulting in bulging discs.

➢ **Long,** or overly flexible, hamstrings can cause instability in the pelvis or knee joints, and are more vulnerable to tears at their origin, the sitz bones.

Gluteal Group

This muscle group comprises both superficial and deep muscles that create the power and base of the spine. The *external rotators* are larger in size and number, and thus are more powerful than the *internal rotators*. They include the *gluteus maximus*, deep and superficial portions, the *piriformis* muscle, and the smaller *obturators* and *gemelli*. The two small internal rotators are the *gluteus minimus* and the anterior section of the *gluteus medius*.

Gluteus Maximus

The *gluteus maximus* gives the buttocks its shape, extends the leg, and is the leg's primary external rotator. The muscle begins on the lateral edge of the sacrum and posterior crest of the ilium, then attaches in a broad band to both the upper section of the posterior thigh bone as well as the posterior side of the IT band, or *iliotibial tract*.

Gluteus Medius

The *gluteus medius* is the primary abductor of the leg (draws the leg away from the midline). When this muscle is at a healthy length, it also prevents the head of the femur bone from drifting away from the midline by forming its boundary. Long or short, when this muscle is out of balance, it can lead to gait disturbance, hip or knee pain, and sacral instability. The muscle originates from the crest of the ilium beneath the gluteus maximus and inserts at the top of the outer thighbone.

➢ A **short** gluteus medius muscle will pull the side of the thigh closer to the hip, making one leg appear shorter than the other.

➢ **Long** muscles allow the heads of the femur bones to wobble away from the midline, destabilizing the pelvis, and compromising our ability to balance on one leg.

Piriformis Muscle

The *piriformis* is another primary external rotator of the leg; in approximately 30 percent of the population, the sciatic nerve passes through the center of the muscle. In fact, sciatica could at times be more correctly understood as Spastic Piriformis Syndrome.

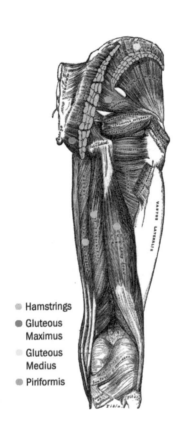

● Hamstrings
● Gluteous Maximus
● Gluteous Medius
● Piriformis

➤ **Short** external rotators cause the feet to turn out, like duck feet, and combine with short hamstrings to prevent the pelvis from tipping forward in a forward bend. The low back will round severely instead, becoming weak over time and vulnerable to injury.

➤ **Long** external rotators will show posturally as knock-knees, or as instability in the posterior pelvic floor and sacrum. Sacral instability is its own form of back and hip pain, most often experienced by women.

Hip Flexors

The *hip flexors* are the group of muscles that pull your thigh forward and help to raise the thighbone when you walk or run. Many hours of sitting shortens these muscles, compromising your ability to stand up straight.

Quadriceps (Quads)

The *quadriceps* run from the hip to below the knee, and they flex the leg and extend/straighten the knee.

Iliopsoas and Iliacus

The *iliopsoas* and *iliacus* are also known as our core, or main postural, muscles. They connect the back body to the front body, and the top to the bottom. They run from inside the back bottom ribs to the front pelvis at the inner groin, and they lie deep inside behind the organs. They create the curves of the spine, flex the leg toward the spine, flex the spine toward the leg, and stabilize the pelvis when we're sitting.

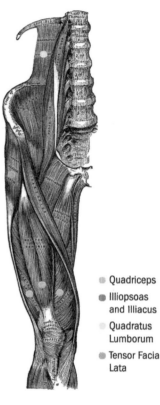

● Quadriceps

● Iliopsoas and Iliacus

○ Quadratus Lumborum

● Tensor Facia Lata

➤ **Short** hip flexor muscles will cause someone to stand with the pelvis tipped forward as if the person were sitting. The top thighs will be pulled forward and the body will present a *swayback* or an accentuated lumbar curve. A deep lumbar curve can cause compression in the facet joints in that area, irritating the nerves and causing back pain. Deeper investigation will reveal the head of the femur bone also pulled forward in the socket, so when that person lies flat, their thighbones will pop up off the floor.

➤ **Long** hip flexor muscles yield a long, soft belly, a sense of the thighbones dropping straight down out of the pelvis, and a more upright spine from the front hip crease up to the nipple region. If these muscles are too long, there will not be enough muscle tone to stabilize the front of the spine making the back muscles contract and overwork, leading to back pain.

Quadratus Lumborum

The *quadratus lumborum* is a deep posterior trunk muscle, arising from the crest of the hip and inserting on the 12th rib and along the lumbar spine. These muscles control or contribute to your ability to bend to the side, lift, and twist. This muscle is listed here for ease of viewing along with the hip flexors.

➤ A **short** or spastic quadratus lumborum muscle causes the spine to bend sideways, or the hip to rise up, undoing the balance of the clock face and the pelvic floor. If and when one side is shortened, the opposite side will become long.

➤ A **long** quadratus lumborum muscle also tends to reflect the loss of the lumbar curve.

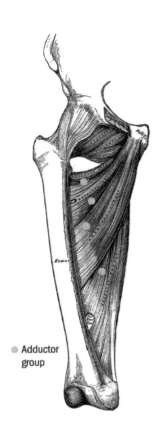

● Adductor
group

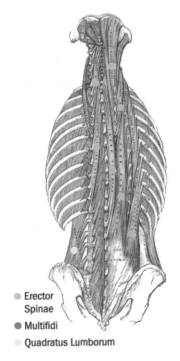

● Erector
Spinae

● Multifidi

○ Quadratus Lumborum

Adductors of the Legs

The seven muscles of the inner leg are large and powerful. They draw the leg in toward the centerline, which creates stability. The *adductors* originate on the pubis and ischium bones and insert mainly on the inside posterior surface of the femur.

➤ **Short** leg adductors narrow the spacing of the pelvic floor, also narrowing the anterior lumbar spine. For added and necessary space in the front of the pelvis and lumbar, the adductors or inner legs need to be lengthened. Short adductors also cause the head of the femur bone to be misaligned in the socket, leading to degeneration and spurs in the hip joint.

➤ **Long** adductors are rare, but in the case that a person has long or weak inner leg muscles, it would be characterized by a wide pelvic floor and possible instability in the hip joints.

Back Muscles

The back muscles form the main support for all movements of the spine, including bending, flexing, and twisting. The largest low back muscle is mentioned first, reserving discussion of the upper back muscles for the anatomy of the shoulders section on page 67.

Latissimus Dorsi

I call these the *cape muscles*, because they wrap around the back like a cape. They originate at the sixth thoracic vertebra and span down to the sacrum. They fan around the body and attach on the upper front surface of the arms under the deltoids. They are the muscles of dynamic movement, and they initiate extension of the arms. (See the image at the top of the next page and page 67.)

➤ **Short** muscles prevent people from raising their arms above their head without the bottom ribs moving forward, causing a deep angle where the arms and shoulders meet. This pulls the lumbar vertebrae forward, which compresses the spine. In this predicament, if and when you stabilize the front ribs, the top arms will be pulled down out of flexion.

➤ **Long** muscles will allow the arms to rise fully above the head without disturbing the plumb line of the hips, ribs, or shoulders. An overly long muscle is not common, as this muscle contracts every time we move our arms; but if it did occur, this could contribute to instability in the lower back.

Erector Spinae and Multifidi Muscles

The *erector spinae* are a group of short and long fibers that overlap to create movement and stability throughout the 26 vertebrae of the spine. The *multifidi* are the deepest back muscles that attach the vertebrae above to the one below and manage the small movements of the spine. In scoliosis, these muscles are out of balance, with one side stronger than the other, even alternating side to side in different segments, as the spine is spiraling sometimes in two directions.

➤ **Short** erector spinae muscles cause a lack of flexibility along the spine and limit mobility of the torso. This presents as difficulty twisting, rounding forward, or bending backward.

➤ **Long** muscles result in an unstable spine with too much mobility, which is therefore vulnerable to strain.

Note: *The erector spinae muscles, along with the psoas major, form a system of four muscular bundles arranged around and supporting the front and back of the lumbar spine like four flexible pillars.*

Abdominal Muscles

People often think they need to have six-pack abs in order to be considered strong and healthy. However, that is not necessarily the case. Each abdominal muscle needs a balance of flexibility and tone like any other muscle.

Rectus Abdominis

Rectus abdominis, the actual six-pack muscles, are the most superficial abdominal muscles, and they connect the pubic bone to the bottoms of ribs 5–7 and the tip of the sternum.

➢ **Short** or overly toned muscles will tend to pull down on the front ribs, inhibiting the free flow of breath and limiting the extension of the front of the spine. The inability to extend the spine causes compression on the front of the discs and rigidity, which increases the likelihood that a disc may herniate.

➢ **Long** rectus abdominus muscles diminish the support for the front of the spine, causing compression and discomfort in the facet joints as gravity pulls the abdominal organs forward. Typically, post-partum women have loose abdominal muscles, leaving their backs vulnerable to strain until muscle tone returns.

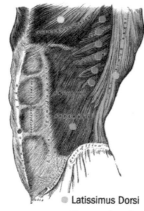

- Latissimus Dorsi
- Serratus Anterior
- Pectoralis Major
- External Obliques

Internal and External Obliques

The *internal* and *external obliques* are the muscles that form the side body, and they are considered part of the abdominal muscle group. They contract in lifting and twisting movements.

➢ **Short** muscles pull and compress the ribs more strongly to one side, contributing to a side tilt. Short muscles occur on one side as the result of an injury, or as a result of the dominant use of one side.

➢ **Long** muscles allow the abdominal organs to expand and the side body to lose tone. When the muscles of one side are short, however toning the longer side will help relieve and balance the short side.

Note: *Both the quadratus lumborum and the obliques are involved in a lifting or twisting injury. Habitual movement such as leg crossing will likely present as one hip higher than the other, or the rib cage on one side will be pulled down. Muscular imbalance leaves us more susceptible to an injury. (See Hip Flexors.)*

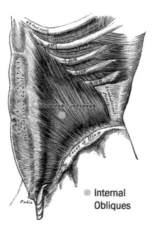

- Internal Obliques

Transverse Abdominis

The *transverse abdominis* comprise the deepest layer of abdominal muscles. They're made of strong horizontal fibers. Known as the *girdle* or *coughing muscle*, this layer connects the anterior crest of the hips to ribs 7–12, wrapping from back to front. They're located beneath the other three abdominal muscles, the rectus abdominis, and the internal and external obliques.

➢ **Long** muscles are common in a forward tilted pelvis and pelvic instability. Watch for the prolapse of the lower abdominal organs and lack of support for the lower back. Also, there will be an inability to draw in and lift the center of the clock face of the pelvic floor, and maintain the lift.

➢ **Short** muscles present as an overly tight lower abdomen, possibly contributing to infertility.

Note: *The importance of this muscle cannot be overemphasized, as its tone offers primary support to the lower back by drawing the abdominal organs in and up also activating the length of the psoas muscle.*

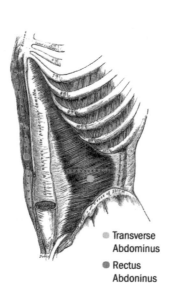

- Transverse Abdominus
- Rectus Abdoninus

Diaphragm

The *diaphragm* is the primary respiration muscle. It's dome-shaped and sits above the abdominal organs, attaching circularly to the lower six ribs and the lumbar vertebrae.

➢ **Short** diaphragm muscles restrict a person's ability to breath deeply. When both the diaphragm and the rectus abdominis are short, the front chest may be anchored down, preventing upright posture.

➢ **Long** diaphragm muscles are unlikely, except perhaps in a disease process.

The Arches of the Feet

The following muscles, despite not being in or near the back, are very important to back health because the feet control the hips, and the hips and legs extend the spine. These muscles form the arches in your feet, which support the lift of the pelvic floor, and thus helping lift the spine from its base.

Anterior Tibialis

The *anterior tibialis* muscle connects to the front upper portion of the tibia or shin bone and runs down the outer calf, across the front of the ankle, and under the first toe. This is the primary muscle of the foot's inner arch.

➢ **Long** muscles present as a collapsed inner arch, with the inner knee turning back and the outer shin rolled forward.

➢ **Short** muscles cause a high inner arch and a collapsed outer arch.

Peroneus Longus and Brevis

The *peroneus longus* and *brevis* muscles run along the outside of the leg from below the knee, behind the outer ankle, and under the foot, inserting on the big toe. This muscle presses the big toe down and creates the outer arch.

➢ **Short** muscles flatten the inner arch of the foot.

➢ **Long** muscles weaken and sometimes collapse the outer ankle.

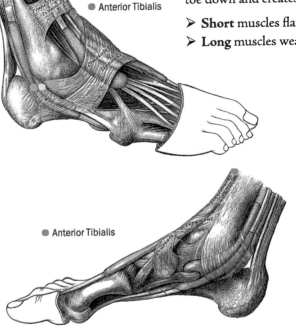

● Peronius Longus
○ Peronius Brevis
● Anterior Tibialis

● Anterior Tibialis

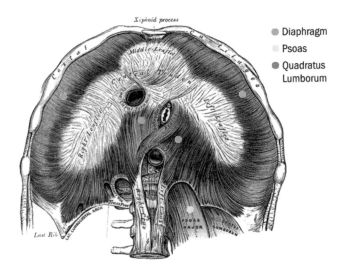

● Diaphragm
○ Psoas
● Quadratus Lumborum

Basic Low Back Sequence

To start your journey toward back pain relief, practice the sequence presented here. If you feel uncertain about performing all 12 exercises, I recommend you begin with the **first four**, adding one more each week until you can do all 12. The first six poses are intended to release tight muscles and begin creating length and space in your spine, and the remaining poses will help you build the strength you need to stabilize your low back, thus continuing to reduce your back pain.

As you practice each yoga pose presented, begin to observe where your muscles are particularly stiff and where they're looser. By building awareness of your body with its particular strengths and weaknesses, you'll be able to then choose the right poses for your condition to create improved muscular balance and more lasting pain relief.

Select a minimum of three days this week to perform this 30-minute practice. Pick a specific time to practice on each of those days and **write it in your schedule.** Follow the same routine for three weeks. When time is at a premium, I recommend practicing the 12–minute "short form" sequence on page 144, rather than skip a practice.

Choose a quiet place and a time when you know you'll be undisturbed. Slow down, breathe deeply, stretch, tune in, and get to know your body better. Observe and find out which stretches are the most helpful to you. As you get familiar with your body, spend more time in the poses that offer you the most relief. If you're particularly stiff, try exercising after a hot shower, or use your exercises as a time to unwind and refresh at the end of the day.

If you currently have a regular exercise or workout routine and are having back pain, I suggest you discontinue those exercises for 7–10 days and practice the Basic Low Back Sequence instead. Observe your results, and then gradually reintroduce your other exercises one or two at a time. Sometimes weak muscles may get stiff and sore from the new exercises. If your discomfort lasts more than three days, discontinue the exercise in question; after two weeks, see if you can add it back in, and/or seek professional guidance.

POSE 1. TRACTION TWIST / SUPTA MATSYANGASANA

This pose offers a gentle beginning to your practice to warm and lengthen the psoas muscles.

➤**1.** Place both feet on the floor, wider than your hips. ➤**2.** Drop your knees to the left so that your right knee is in line with your nose. Your pelvis will lift up about halfway. ➤**3.** Extend from your outer right hip toward your knee, as you curl your tail in. ➤**4.** Inhale, pause, and as you exhale, drop your navel in and draw it up towards your ribs. Feel the stretch on your top thigh. ➤**5.** Keep your knee steady as you turn your waist back toward the floor any amount. ➤**6.** Hold for 3–5 breaths on each side. Repeat.

Hint: Protect your knee by flexing your foot and drawing the toes back toward your shin.

CAUTION: If your right knee suffers any discomfort, please honor that and place a block under the knee to support it both above and below the joint. If any knee pain persists, stop doing the pose.

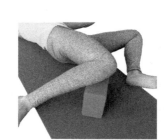

POSE 2. **ALTERNATE KNEE-TO-CHEST / APANASANA**

This pose continues to warm and lengthen the psoas muscles.

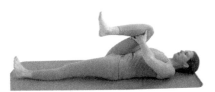

➤**1.** Lie on your back with your legs out straight. ➤**2.** Draw your right knee toward your armpit chest, holding behind the knee with both hands. ➤**3.** Drop 6:00 toward the floor to press the straight leg down and keep your clock face balanced. ➤**4.** As you exhale, slowly draw your right knee closer to your side chest while pressing the straight left leg down and out along the floor. Back off the stretch as you inhale; draw in as you exhale. ➤**5.** Change legs. Repeat and hold for 3–5 breaths on each side.

Hint: Roll the straight leg in until the foot and knee are vertical.

CAUTION: Keep your straight leg heel on the floor as you press the thigh down in order to anchor the whole leg and maintain the stretch of the psoas muscle.

POSE 3. **STRAP STRETCH I / SUPTA PADANGUSTHASANA**

This pose stretches the hamstrings and indirectly releases tension in the low back muscles.

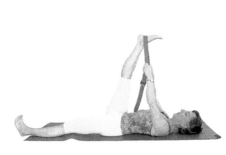

➤**1.** Lie on your back. Bend your right knee and place a strap across the back of the arch for more stability to easily hold the weight of the leg. Hold onto the ends of the strap with both hands. ➤**2.** Straighten your right leg and extend your arms toward your raised foot, elbows straight, keeping your shoulder blades flat on the floor. ➤**3.** Raise the right leg up as high as you can without bending the knee. Breathe. ➤**4.** Press your left inner thigh down toward the floor and extend the leg out through your heel. ➤**5.** When you exhale, extend the right heel toward the ceiling; as you inhale, draw down from the back of your knee to the floor. ➤**6.** Maintain the balance of your clock face by moving the right hip away from your waist and toward the opposite inner thigh. ➤**7.** As the muscles loosen, your raised foot will move slowly toward your head. ➤**8.** Hold the pose for 5–7 breaths, or up to 1 minute. ➤**9.** Lower the right leg and feel the difference between the legs. ➤**10.** Repeat this exercise with the left leg raised.

Hint: Maintain the normal curve in your lower back by keeping your pelvic clock parallel to the floor and level; i.e., drop 6:00 toward the floor and lower the leg as needed to maintain the curve.

POSE 4. **STRAP STRETCH III / SUPTA PADANGUSTHASANA III**

This pose will stretch the muscles of the outer hip and thigh, as well as lengthen the sides of your waist, decompressing the lower back one side at a time.

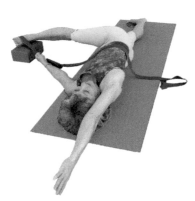

➤**1.** Lie on the floor. Place the strap on the back arch of your right foot, this time holding both ends of the strap in your left hand. ➤**2.** Extend the leg out of the hip and carry it across your body, roll onto the outside of your left hip completely, and rest your foot on the floor or a block. ➤**3.** Straighten both legs and spread the toes. ➤**4.** Extend your right arm alongside your head as you move the right hip away from your waist. Breathe. ➤**5.** Maintain the arch of your lower back by lifting your breastbone toward your chin and extending your left leg. ➤**6.** Extend your right leg any amount more by drawing back on the outer edge of the foot. ➤**7.** Hold this pose for 5–7 breaths, or up to 1 minute, and repeat on the other side.

Hint: Be certain your sacrum is perpendicular to the floor by sliding your hand from the right buttock to the left to see if they're stacked. This will take pressure off the sacroiliac joint and keep the lumbar spine stable.

Hint 2: Draw the inner shoulder blade away from your ears to release your shoulder.

CAUTION: Come out of this pose with a bent knee when necessary to avoid triggering any negative pain in your lower back.

POSE 5. **LOW LUNGE / VANARASANA**

This simple lunge helps lengthen the quadriceps and psoas muscles, an important antidote to too much sitting, which shortens the muscles of the front thigh and groin, contributing to back pain.

➤**1.** Begin on your hands and knees. ➤**2.** Move your left foot forward between your hands to form a 90-degree angle between your calf and thigh (i.e., the center of the ankle should be directly under the knee). ➤**3.** Slide the right leg as far back as possible to extend the front of the rear thigh. ➤**4.** Draw the center of the clock face in and up as you bend the front knee any amount. ➤**5.** Turn the front knee slightly out to draw the outer hip in toward the midline. ➤**6.** Do this for 5–7 breaths on each side.

Hint: Square your pelvis to balance your clock face by placing both edges of the pubic bone parallel to the floor.

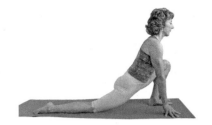

POSE 6. **BOUND ANGLE POSE / BADDHAKONASANA**

The muscles of the inner thighs are large and powerful. Stretching these muscles releases their pull on the front pelvis and low back.

➤**1.** Sit on a blanket with your pelvis tight to the wall. ➤**2.** Bring the bottoms of the feet to touch and open the knees wide. ➤**3.** Lift the top of the sacrum away from the wall to keep from collapsing the low back. ➤**4.** Extend from the inner thighs out beyond the knee, and then draw from the outer knee toward your buttocks. ➤**5.** Lift the bottom of your belly in and up to extend the lumbar spine. ➤**6.** Hold for 7–10 breaths.

Hint: Balance the extension of each inner leg until the knees are the same height by focusing your attention on the tighter side.

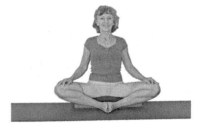

Optional arm extension

➤**1.** Interlace your fingers and turn the palms out. ➤**2.** Extend the arms in front of you and then up on an exhalation. ➤**3.** Keep your front ribs from pushing out. ➤**4.** Lift both sides of the torso from the hips to the ribs. ➤**5.** Switch the interlace of the fingers and repeat. ➤**6.** Hold the arm extension for 3–5 breaths on a side.

Hint: Persons with limited shoulder flexibility may hold a stick with the hands shoulder-width apart.

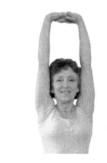

POSE 7. **STAND TALL / TADASANA**

Tadasana is the pose of ideal alignment in relationship to gravity. Practicing this pose helps to build our awareness of balance, as well as align our four diaphragms for greatest postural ease.

➤**1.** Stand with the feet 2 inches apart and parallel. ➤**2.** To lift the inner arch of the foot, bring the inner knee joints forward to face each other, while turning your outer top shins back. ➤**3.** Now lift the outer anklebones so the weight is balanced in the center of each foot. ➤**4.** Lift up your inner leg to your pelvic floor, and from the pelvic floor up to your chest. ➤**5.** Lift the bottom of your belly and draw your top buttocks down to flatten your clock face. ➤**6.** Release the heels further down as you float the back bottom ribs up. ➤**7.** Roll the shoulders back and down as you lift the center of your chest high. ➤**8.** Move the base of your head back to find alignment from the top of your head to the front of your heel. ➤**9.** Explore the balance of this pose for 5–7 breaths.

Hint: Stand sideways and look in a mirror to see if your top thighs are back far enough for your pelvic floor to be in line with the crown of your head. Also look to see that your pelvic and respiratory diaphragms are parallel to the ground. Observe which muscles are contracting to hold you in balance.

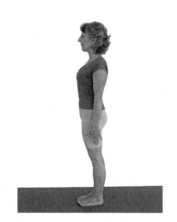

POSE 8. **SIDE STRETCH / ARDHA CHANDRASANA I**

To create length and space in the spine, we also need to elongate the muscles of the side body, including the small muscles that lie between each rib by applying this pose.

➤**1.** Begin Standing Erect with the feet square and hip-width apart. ➤**2.** Clasp your elbows above your head. ➤**3.** Inhale and extend your elbows up from your waist. ➤**4.** Keeping your lower belly lifted and your hips drawn back above your ankles and stable, tilt to one side. ➤**5.** Inhale, move back to center, exhale, and tilt again. ➤**6.** Repeat 3 times on each side. Change sides. ➤**7.** Total time for each side is 3–5 breaths.

Hint: Extend the length of your side body evenly from your hips to your armpit area. Observe the differences on each side. When one side is significantly shorter, spend a bit more time extending that side.

POSE 9. **LATERAL LEG LIFT / UTTHITA MERUDANDASANA**

This is the first of several poses that tone rather than stretch muscles. Here, the side muscles of the outer thigh, hip, and waist are made stronger. The pose also tones the inner thigh of the lower leg.

➤**1.** Lie on your right side, with the elbow of the bottom arm straight out, head resting on the arm. ➤**2.** Place your left arm 10 inches out from the center of your chest to form a tripod for balance. ➤**3.** Extend the back of the knees down toward your heels and up toward your buttocks, tightening the knees completely. ➤**4.** Lift the bottom of your belly in and up to stabilize and extend your spine and flatten your clock face. ➤**5.** Now raise both legs off the floor 6–8 inches without rolling the hips forward or back. ➤**6.** Continue by lifting the top leg 4 inches higher, and then lower the top leg back to the bottom leg. Repeat 3–5 times. ➤**7.** Put both legs down. Change sides, and then repeat each side again.

Hint: As you raise your legs, lead with your heels in order to access the sides of your hip and waist directly.

POSE 10. **LOCUST POSE / SALABHASANA**

This is a foundational pose for strengthening the lower back. I recommend elevating the hips on a blanket or a bolster, as shown in the photograph, to protect the low back from pinching.

➤**1.** Lie on your stomach, fold a blanket (or use a bolster), and place it under the front of your pelvis. ➤**2.** Curl the toes under and lift the inner knees and inner thighs up away from the floor. ➤**3.** Extend your legs back firmly. ➤**4.** Press your pelvis into the blanket, keeping your inner thighs lifted. ➤**5.** Extend from your navel to the center of your chest to lengthen your front spine. ➤**6.** Roll your shoulders back as you bring your breastbone forward. ➤**7.** Lift your chest and shoulders any amount, keeping your feet pressing down on the floor. ➤**8.** Reach your legs back and your breastbone forward to curl your spine. ➤**9.** Draw your sitting bones toward your feet and press your armpit chest forward any amount. ➤**10.** Repeat the pose 3–5 times, holding 3–5 breaths each time.

Hint: In the beginning, less is more. Pay attention to curl the spine evenly from top to bottom, no matter how high you lift, so that the sensation of lifting is distributed along your spine.

CAUTION: Lift only as far as you are able without pinching the tube of your spine in the lower back. Listen and feel. If you have any negative pain in your lower back, firm your legs, drop your tail, lengthen the front of your spine, but don't lift!

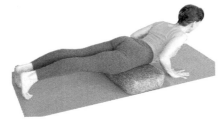

POSE 11. **KNEELING GROIN STRETCH / ARDHA MANDUKASANA**

This is an excellent first-aid pose to help relieve lower back fatigue or pain, and you can practice it on its own as needed.

➤**1.** From a kneeling position, spread your knees wide apart, keeping your toes touching as much as possible. ➤**2.** Place your elbows on the floor under your shoulders. ➤**3.** Position the hips near your knees so you can easily flatten your lower back. ➤**4.** Keep your clock face parallel to the floor. ➤**5.** Feel free to move your hips slowly forward and back to release the tension in your inner legs. ➤**6.** Hold the position for 5–7 breaths.

Hint: To relieve mid-back pain, take your elbows forward and out to the side. Rest your forehead or chin on your hands. Allow your chest to drop down and your spine to curve in.

POSE 12. **YOGI CURL-UPS**

Strengthening the abdominal muscles is one of the first defenses to stabilize the low back. In this position, toning the abdominals also employs "reciprocal inhibition" to release any muscle tightness in the low back, returning the spine to neutral.

➤**1.** Lie on your back with your knees bent and your feet on the floor, hip-width apart. ➤**2.** Cross your arms behind your head, touching each shoulder with the opposite hand, or simply hold your elbows in front of your chest as in Pose 1A of Progressive Abdominal Toning on page 33. ➤**3.** On an exhale, raise your head, shoulders, and chest off the floor one-third of the way, keeping the bottom back ribs touching the floor. ➤**4.** Keep your inner thighs soft and your chin off your chest. ➤**5.** Gaze at your knees and breathe. ➤**6.** Hold for 3–5 breaths; release and rest your head, chest, and arms on the floor. ➤**7.** Repeat 3 times.

Hint: For a more complete softening of the inner groin, rest your calves on a chair seat, or place your feet on a wall, calves and thighs at a 90-degree angle as in Pose 2 of the Basic Neck and Shoulder Sequence on page 29.

POSE 13. **CORPSE POSE / SAVASANA**

Choose one of the two following options for relaxation at the end of your practice. This is important to do so your muscles and nerves have time to restore and integrate the changes you have asked for.

Version A—Suspended Relaxation

➤**1.** Fold one blanket lengthwise about 6–8 inches wide. ➤**2.** Place the narrow edge of the blanket at the back of your waist, and lie down so your ribcage is lifted. ➤**3.** Place a second folded blanket under your head as a small pillow, with the back of the neck supported. ➤**4.** Elevate the lower legs with the calves and feet resting on a bolster, knees bent and turned out. ➤**5.** Use your hands to lift your buttocks and move the flesh toward your feet so your lower back lengthens and your hips rest evenly on the floor. ➤**6.** Turn your palms up and draw your inner shoulder blades away from your ears. ➤**7.** Stay in this position for 5 minutes. ➤**8.** Breathe easy.

Version B—Relaxation with Calves on a Chair

➤**1.** With your back flat on the floor, place your calves on the seat of a chair. ➤**2.** Place the middle of the back of your knees at the edge of the chair seat. ➤**3.** Let your calves rest heavy. ➤**4.** Stay in this position for 5 minutes.

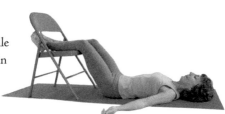

Hint: For a deeper rest and more relief for low back spasms, place a 10-pound bag of rice or other substance across your lower abdomen.

Basic Neck and Shoulder Sequence

Due to gravity and the dynamics of movement, the human spine works as a system. Therefore, what affects the lower back also has an effect on the mid and upper back, the neck and shoulders, and vise versa. The sequence presented here complements the Basic Low Back Sequence, helping to not only relieve pain in the neck and shoulders, but to contribute to greater overall ease of movement through the whole spine.

With the onset of the computer age, challenges to the arms and hands are at an all time high. In order to maintain the healthy function of the arms and thumbs that we rely upon, it's important to maintain the flexibility of the shoulders. Our head, hands, and arms host 80 percent of the nerve endings in our bodies. When we stretch, our overly contracted muscles, tendons, and fascia may pinch the tube of some nerves. Be mindful to seek out positive pain and avoid practicing in a way that may cause any fingers to tingle or go numb.

However, if you experience tingling or numbness in your arms while performing the poses presented in this sequence, remember the guidance of a good yoga practice: when you meet the resistance, Stop, Wait, Breathe, Suspend Judgment, and back off 10 percent. Also, test the poses by going in and out of the stretch for short periods of time, choosing compassionate listening before holding the poses longer. The ultimate test of positive action is the sense of relief and freedom you experience when you finish a pose. Again, select three days this week to perform this 30–40 minute practice. Pick a specific time and write it in your schedule. Follow the same routine for three weeks. You will find a recommended "short form" on page 145 that can be done in 11–12 minutes when time is at a premium and you need quick relief.

Observe and find out which stretches are the most helpful to you. As you get familiar with your body, spend more time in the poses that offer you the most relief. As time progresses, try practicing the Basic Low Back and the Basic Neck and Shoulder Sequence on alternate days.

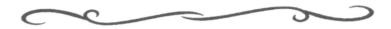

POSE 1. **BASIC LYING TWIST / JATHARA PARIVARTANASANA**

Arm circles done lying down will soften and release tension in all the muscles of the shoulder and neck.

➤**1.** Lie on your back, legs straight out, with your arms out to the side, palms face up. ➤**2.** Bend your knees and draw them toward your chest. ➤**3.** Roll over the crest of your hip and carry your knees to the right. Rest your knees and feet on a stack of one or two folded blankets or block. ➤**4.** Reach out with your left arm and describe a half circle down past your right hip to your right hand. ➤**5.** Keep your neck relaxed and extend your left arm out from the shoulder as if it were a solid tube until both palms touch. ➤**6.** Continue sweeping the arm over your head along the floor to finish the second half of the circle back to the starting position, keeping your elbow straight. ➤**7.** Repeat making 3 full circles in one direction and then reverse directions for 3 full circles. ➤**8.** Pull your knees in toward your chest and back to center. Change sides.

Hint: Be certain the knees are closer to your chest than your navel to elongate and release the lower spine.

CAUTION 1: If you feel any strain in your low back, lessen the twist by raising your knees higher by adding a block or an additional blanket for support so you can focus on releasing the neck and shoulders.

CAUTION 2: If your shoulders are particularly tight, you may not be able to touch the floor above your head. In that case, simply allow your arm to float above the floor. Find the place of stability and ease.

POSE 2. **YOGI CURL-UPS**

Tone the abdominal, upper psoas, and scalene muscles of the front neck, while releasing tension in the upper back and neck. This is a good example of "Reciprocal Inhibition."

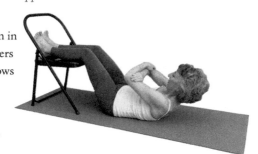

➤**1.** Lie on your back, bend your knees, and place your calves on the seat of a chair, as shown in the photo. ➤**2.** Cross your arms in front of your chest. ➤**3.** Exhale and curl your shoulders and chest up one third of the way keeping the bottom back ribs on the floor, with the elbows extending toward your knees. ➤**4.** Keep your inner groins soft and your eyes gazing at your knees. ➤**5.** Hold for 10 counts, breathing smoothly, and repeat 3 times.

Note: This version of Yogi Curl-Ups is interchangeable with the Basic Low Back version, Pose 12 on page 27 where the feet are on the floor.

POSE 3. **SUPINE HEAD LIFTS**

Holding your head up both strengthens the muscles of the front and releases the muscles of the back of your neck.

➤**1.** Lie on your back, arms out to your side, palms face up. ➤**2.** Bring your feet together and point your toes up. ➤**3.** Exhale and lift your head to gaze at your toes. ➤**4.** Keep your shoulders relaxed. ➤**5.** Hold for 10 counts, and then rest. ➤**6.** Repeat 3 times. ➤**7.** Repeat this exercise one more time, turning your head right for 5 counts, back to center, and then to the left for 5 counts. Don't forget to breathe!

Hint: Holding your head up in this manner may cause some trembling and sensations of pain in the back of your neck. Remember the principle of reciprocal inhibition, and know that those sensations represent tension leaving those muscles.

CAUTION: When turning your head, always deliberately return to the center before lowering your head to avoid unnecessary strain. If your neck feels weak, opt to do one side at a time, resting for 2 breaths in between sides.

POSE 4. **HALF FISH / ARDHA MATSYASANA**

This simple pose helps you connect to and tone the back of the neck, mid-trapezius, and rhomboid muscles building the strength necessary to hold your shoulders back without effort as well as release the tight muscles of the chest through reciprocal inhibition.

➤**1.** Lie on your back with your knees partially bent and your feet resting on the floor hip-width apart. ➤**2.** Bend your elbows and place them 8–10 inches away from your ribs on the floor. ➤**3.** Turn your upper arms completely out until the shoulder blades lie flat against the floor. ➤**4.** Lift your chin until the back of your crown is in contact with the floor. ➤**5.** Press the back of your head and elbows down to engage the muscles of your upper back and neck to lift your chest up, forming an even arc from the top of the neck to the bottom of your shoulder blades. ➤**6.** Pressing the outer edge of the elbow firmly into the floor, broaden your collarbones and draw the inner shoulder blades farther away from your neck. ➤**7.** Hold for 3–5 breaths. Repeat 3 times.

Hint: Pin the bottom tip of your shoulder blades firmly into your back ribs to lift them.

CAUTION: Be sensitive to the back of your neck—sometimes less is more. It's better to lift your chin only 1 inch and create an even arc of the neck, rather than collapse the tube of your neck by throwing your head back too much and risk pinching nerves.

POSE 5. **TRADITIONAL CAT-COW / MARJARYASANA-BITILASANA**

As the body heals through movement, this simple pose not only loosens the whole spine, but also stretches the front and back of the arms at the shoulders, preparing your arms for downward facing dog pose.

➤**1.** Get down on your hands and knees into a tabletop position. ➤**2.** On an exhale, press your back up, curling your tail and tucking your chin, to extend the back of your arms and spine. That's your cat! ➤**3.** On an inhale, arch your back and lift your head, chin, and collarbones as a unit to extend the front of your arms. Here's the cow! ➤**4.** Continue to press the inner palms deeper down to lift the collarbones any amount more. ➤**5.** Reverse directions. ➤**6.** Repeat 5–7 times, coordinating the movement with your breath.

Hint: To receive the most benefit for your neck and shoulders when lifting your head, train yourself to move your collarbones forward and up so the weight comes to the front of your palms.

POSE 6. **DOWNWARD FACING DOG / ADHO MUKHA SVANASANA**

This yoga pose extends the spine by lengthening the arms and the back of the legs. It provides a sense of stability, warming the muscles of the shoulders, while improving circulation in the chest and head.

Feel free to choose either version of downward facing dog pose; first try with the hands on a wall or ledge to learn to evenly extend your spine, and then try the pose with your hands on the floor. The focus of the pose is to extend the spine as an even arc from the back of the neck to the mid sacrum so that no part of the "tube" of the spine is pinched. To accomplish this, the back of the legs will need to lengthen.

Version A

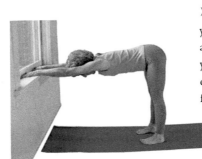

➤**1.** Stand with your feet hip-width apart. ➤**2.** Hinge forward from the front of your hip joint and reach your arms out to touch a wall or a ledge. ➤**3.** Keep your spine long by moving your breastbone forward and your sitz bones back. ➤**4.** Lift your sitz bones any amount to stretch the back of your legs. ➤**5.** Wrap your outer armpit toward the floor and lift the inner arm to release strain in the shoulders. ➤**6.** Keep your ears even with your arms so the weight of your head does not pinch the tube of your shoulders. ➤**7.** Hold for 5–7 breaths.

Hint: Reach your hand behind you to feel your lower back. If you feel the processes of your spine pushing up, you'll need to raise your hands higher up the wall until the normal concave curve of your low back is restored.

Version B

➤**1.** From a kneeling position on your hands and knees, move the palms ahead of your shoulders, and place them with the middle fingers running parallel to each other. ➤**2.** Lift your collarbones as you did in the cat/cow pose. ➤**3.** Squeeze your elbows in. ➤**4.** Move your pubic bone back between your legs to lift your hips up into the pose. ➤**5.** Wrap your outer armpit toward the floor and lift the inner arm to release strain in the shoulders. ➤**6.** Keep your knees bent, and then press the full surface of your palms into the floor to lift and extend your spine farther back and up toward your sitting bones. Keep your heels lifted as you straighten your knees. ➤**7.** Reach the fingers forward as you press the top thighs back to continue extending your spine. ➤**8.** Hold for 5–7 breaths. Repeat 3 times.

Hint: Practice this pose with your hands on a counter or wall when the hamstrings are short. Or when your hands are on the floor keep your knees bent to avoid collapsing the tube of the spine.

POSE 7. **LOW LUNGE — HANDS ON KNEE / VANARASANA**

This pose lengthens the quadriceps and psoas muscles—the front thigh. Opening the front thigh and hip creates length through the front of the spine, helping to release the front chest and neck.

➤**1.** Begin in a low lunge as you did in the Basic Low Back Sequence, Pose 5, on page 25. ➤**2.** Keeping your hips square, press down into your front heel and lift the bottom of your belly to raise your hands up onto your knee. ➤**3.** Press your rear shin down as you draw the center of your clock face in and up. ➤**4.** Lift your top chest to relax your shoulders. ➤**5.** Hold for 5–7 breaths and change sides.

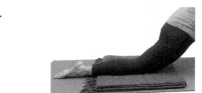

Hint: When raising your hands onto your knee, curl your tail forward to help lift the bottom of your belly.
CAUTION: Avoid excess pressure on your knee by placing a blanket under your knee and the full length of your shin.

POSE 8. **ELBOWS ON THE CHAIR / PINCHA MAYURASANA PREP**

Stretch the latisimus dorsi and the small muscles of the outer armpit with this pose. It will help you gain the ability to extend your arms straight overhead. To prepare, place a towel or pad on the seat of the chair.

➤**1.** Kneeling on the floor, place the center back of the elbows on the chair seat, with the upper arms parallel. ➤**2.** Hold a yoga block between your palms, with your fingers pointing up. ➤**3.** Rest your forehead on the chair, and walk your knees and hips back, spine parallel to the floor. ➤**4.** Lengthen your outer armpits by turning them down, as you draw your hips and ribs back. ➤**5.** Breathe. Hold for 5–7 breaths.

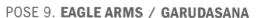

Hint 1: Contain the belly to support the low back as you extend your hips back to release the outer shoulders.
Hint 2: Notice if one shoulder is weaker than the other and place that elbow on the chair first with the block in that hand. Then bring the second hand and elbow into position.

POSE 9. **EAGLE ARMS / GARUDASANA**

This pose stretches the short muscles on the back of the arm and the muscles across the top of the shoulders, releasing tension from the back of the neck.

➤**1.** Sit in a chair, with your back straight. ➤**2.** Hold your arms in front of your chest at right angles. ➤**3.** Cross the left arm under the right at the elbow. Keep the right palm facing left. ➤**4.** Wrap the right palm around to the little finger side of the left hand. ➤**5.** Touch your right palm to the left palm (or fingers). ➤**6.** With the upper arms parallel to the floor, extend the elbows forward to release between the shoulder blades. ➤**7.** Breathe and soften the back of your neck. ➤**8.** Now reverse direction, drawing the elbows toward you. ➤**9.** Drop your shoulder blades and lift your breastbone, keeping your elbows lifted. ➤**10.** Switch the arm on top, and repeat. ➤**11.** Hold for 5–7 breaths on each side.

Hint: If your shoulders are very tight, you may not be able to wrap your hands as shown. In this case, simply keep the palms facing away from each other, and press the forearms against each other where they do touch.

POSE 10. **COW'S HEAD ARMS / GOMUKHASANA**

This pose loosens both the back of the top arm and the front of the lower arm, creating more ease of movement in the shoulder joint itself.

➤**1.** Sit or stand comfortably with your spine straight. ➤**2.** Place your left arm behind you, with the outer wrist against your spine at the level of your waist. ➤**3.** Roll your shoulder forward, up, back, and down, while pointing your elbow out to the side. ➤**4.** Lift your breastbone. ➤**5.** Take your right arm up alongside your head and turn your palm to face back. ➤**6.** Drop your top hand down to grab the opposite fingers, or hold a strap between your hands. ➤**7.** Raise your left ribs as you lower your right in order to breathe evenly into both sides of your chest, balancing the "tube" of your chest. ➤**8.** Hold for 5–7 breaths on each side.

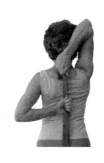

Hint: Press the wrist of the lower hand into your back to help you pin that shoulder blade to your back ribs.

POSE 11. **SIDEWAYS CHAIR TWIST / BHARADVAJASANA**

Twisting motions help to loosen the spine and shoulders by increasing the mobility of the small muscles of the ribs and chest. Using the chair will help you to create length in your spine in order to twist safely.

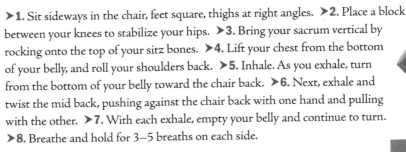

➤**1.** Sit sideways in the chair, feet square, thighs at right angles. ➤**2.** Place a block between your knees to stabilize your hips. ➤**3.** Bring your sacrum vertical by rocking onto the top of your sitz bones. ➤**4.** Lift your chest from the bottom of your belly, and roll your shoulders back. ➤**5.** Inhale. As you exhale, turn from the bottom of your belly toward the chair back. ➤**6.** Next, exhale and twist the mid back, pushing against the chair back with one hand and pulling with the other. ➤**7.** With each exhale, empty your belly and continue to turn. ➤**8.** Breathe and hold for 3–5 breaths on each side.

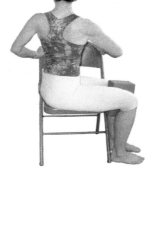

Hint: Lift your spine with each inhale before twisting to decompress the tube of your spine. Know that each vertebrae turns about 2 percent, therefore think to turn incrementally from the base of your spine up.

CAUTION: Adjust the chair to match your height. When sitting in the chair look to see if the center of your hip joint is even with or slightly higher than the center of your knee joint. Place one or more folded blankets on the seat of the chair until you feel the ease of lift in your spine. If you're short, place the blanket under your feet so you have a firm foundation.

POSE 12. **DOOR CHEST HANG / PURVOTTANASANA**

The door chest hang helps to stretch the large pectoralis muscles of the front chest and arms, bringing the chest to a more fully upright position.

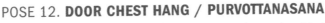

➤**1.** Stand in the center of a doorway. ➤**2.** Hook your fingers around the door jam behind you, placing the base of the palms so they press out on the inner door. ➤**3.** Bring your armpit chest forward and up as you roll your shoulders back and down. ➤**4.** Lift your navel in and up to lift your chest. ➤**5.** Breathe into the upper chest to stretch the upper portion of the front chest and shoulder. ➤**6.** Hold for 5–7 breaths.

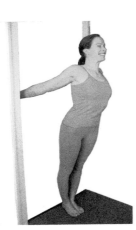

Hint: To increase the stretch, walk your feet forward 3–4 inches, and/or raise your hands up any amount.

CAUTION: If you experience any numbness in your arms, back off 10 percent by lowering your hands, and breathe deeply. Sometimes less is more. Check to see that your top shoulder is rolled back and the bottom tips of the shoulder blades are pinned to your back ribs.

POSE 13. **CORPSE POSE / SAVASANA**

In this version of corpse pose gravity and slow relaxed deep breathing will release the tension in the small muscles of the front shoulder just below the collar bones and the sides of the neck.

Variation C: Over a blanket

➤**1.** Fold a blanket lengthwise (6–8 inches wide) and place it horizontally on the floor. ➤**2.** Lay your shoulders on the blanket, arms out to the side and head on the floor. ➤**3.** Turn the upper arms completely out, palms up. ➤**4.** Keep the bottom of the shoulder blades caught on the blanket. ➤**5.** With your knees bent, push your chest back until it curls over the blanket. ➤**6.** Straighten your legs and rest for 5 minutes.

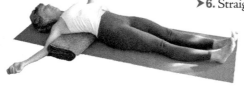

Abdominal Progressions for Back Care

The poses in this section exercise all the abdominal muscles: the iliopsoas, rectus abdominis, transverse abdominis, internal and external obliques, and the scalene muscles of the front neck. I have organized them to begin with the most basic versions that are appropriate for persons experiencing some level of back pain. I offer two or more versions of most of the poses, again working from basic to more difficult.

When you're experiencing back pain, begin with Pose 1, Version A. Always keep the center of your pelvic clock face in place and make your belly feel hollow by pulling the center point of the clock down onto the floor, which will begin to tone your transverse abdominus (see anatomy information on page 21). When you finish the pose, the measure of your success will be a feeling of relief, without any back pain. Once you experience that, add the basic versions of Pose 2 and Pose 3 to your routine. Build your muscle tone gradually, which will eventually give you access to all the small muscle fibers that have remained weak in the past.

No one is expected to perform all of these poses at one time, nor a variation of each pose in one session. Rather, start with the basics and build up to include one, two, or three abdominal poses each time you practice. As you progress toward more challenging versions, you'll find your abdominal tone and stability improving.

Hold each pose to your capacity. Listen to your body—be your own best friend. When you start to quiver or shake, the muscles are showing signs of fatigue. Better to hold for several short rounds than overexert for one long round. I recommend repeating each pose you choose to do three times. Also, you'll find the poses listed here peppered throughout the book and you can interchange them.

When practicing all these poses, remember that alignment principles always apply. Please be mindful to keep the toes and knees pointing straight up when the legs are extended, and attend to the horizontal and vertical balance of the pelvic clock.

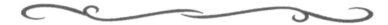

POSE 1. YOGI CURL-UPS

This pose tones the transverse abdominus and only the upper fibers of the psoas muscles, keeping the lower back neutral. Version C also tones the oblique abdominal muscles. Lie on your back with your knees bent and your feet on the floor, hip-width apart. Or you can place your feet on a wall or chair with your legs at right angles for more release in the low back. Start by doing either Version A or B, and then do Version C.

Version A

➤**1.** Hold your elbows in front of your chest. ➤**2.** On an exhale, curl up one third of the way. Keep your chin neutral, and gaze at your knees.

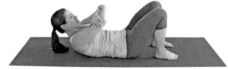

Version B

➤**1.** Cross your arms behind your head for additional neck support, with each hand touching the opposite shoulder. ➤**2.** On an exhale, curl up one third of the way. Keep your chin neutral, and gaze at your knees.

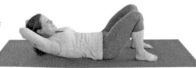

Version C—Curl-up with a twist

➤**1.** With your arms in either position from Version A or B, on an exhale curl up one third of the way.
➤**2.** Add a twist by bringing the left shoulder toward your right knee, and hold here for a couple of breaths. Repeat the twist on the other side by bringing your right shoulder toward the left knee, and hold. Observe which side seems weak, and hold that position longer, perhaps 5–7 breaths.

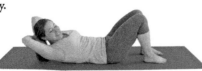

Hint: Keep your inner groin soft, feet grounded. Breathe by expanding your side ribs.

POSE 2. **ALTERNATE KNEES TO CHEST / APANASANA**

Condition your psoas muscle gradually by lifting one leg at a time up and down. This way of practicing uses the weight of the legs to both lengthen and evenly tone the psoas muscles.

➤**1.** Lie flat on your back with your legs out straight. ➤**2.** Draw your right knee into your armpit chest by holding the front of the knee with both hands. Be sure to keep 3:00 and 9:00 level. ➤**3.** Extend the left leg straight out and press it down onto the floor,. ➤**4.** As you inhale, lift the straight left leg up from the floor as high as possible without tilting the clock face. ➤**5.** As you exhale, slowly lower the leg 6–10 inches from the floor, paying special attention to pulling the center of your clock face in and up. ➤**6.** Repeat the straight leg lift 3–6 times. ➤**7.** Change sides and repeat with the other leg drawn into the chest.

Hint: Find the sweet spot for the bent leg by drawing the outer hip toward the opposite thigh and turning your knee to point toward your armpit rather than into your chest.

CAUTION 1: If lifting the straight leg causes any back pain, simply begin by bending and drawing the knee in toward the chest before straightening the leg toward the ceiling. Lower the leg on the exhale and repeat.

CAUTION 2: If you aren't able to lower the leg to 6 inches from the floor while keeping the center of the clock face drawn in and up, only go as far as you can. An option is to place your foot on a tall or medium high block and practice lifting your foot 1 inch off the block by activating the center of your clock face.

POSE 3. **ALTERNATING KNEE CURL-UPS / APANASANA VARIATION**

This way of practicing will intensify the work and tone of all the abdominal muscles while keeping the low back neutral. Use this version to get instant relief from a low back spasm. Begin lying on your back. You may choose to do one or both of the following variations.

Version A

➤**1.** Keep your left foot on the floor and hold onto your right kneecap with both hands. ➤**2.** Press your right knee out to arm's length to create resistance as you draw the center of your clock face in and up. ➤**3.** On an exhale, curl the head and chest up toward the right knee, keeping the knee stationary. ➤**4.** Lift the elbows out and up as you draw the inner shoulders down. ➤**5.** Hold for 3–5 breaths. Change sides. Repeat 3 times.

Version B

➤**1.** Repeat steps 1–4 from Version A. ➤**2.** Bend then extend the left leg straight up and lower it with an exhalation until your foot is 4–10 inches off the floor. ➤**3.** Hold for 3–5 breaths. Change sides. Repeat 3 times.

Hint: Be certain to remain balanced on the center of the clock face as well as to keep drawing the lower belly in and up.

POSE 4. **SUPINE UPPER BACK TWIST / SUPTA MARICHYASANA III**

Although somewhat challenging, this unique pose broadens the space between the shoulder blades, giving horizontal spread and traction to the shoulder joints, as well as deeply toning the psoas and oblique abdominal muscles.

➤**1.** Bend both knees and place your feet on the floor. ➤**2.** Bring one knee in toward your chest and curl up to capture the knee with the opposite elbow (or use a strap loop around the knee to slide your elbow through). ➤**3.** Place the second elbow out to the side for stability and bring your palms together. ➤**4.** Keep the bent knee perpendicular to the floor as you twist the upper body toward the knee. ➤**5.** Keep the clock face stable.

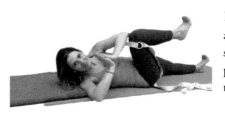

Pose 4 continued next page

Choose one of the two following variations:

Version A

➤**1.** Keep the opposite foot on the floor and your hips and clock face stable. ➤**2.** Hold for 3–5 breaths. Change sides and repeat.

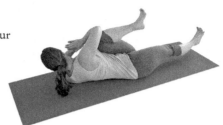

Version B

➤**1.** Straighten the opposite leg and lower it down until you feel the effort to keep your clock face stable, approximately 6–10 inches from the floor. ➤**2.** Keep turning the straight leg groin in so your foot points straight up. ➤**3.** Hold for 3–5 breaths. Change sides and repeat.

Hint: Allow the bent knee to press forward to traction your shoulder away from your neck. Find a neutral position for your neck by gazing toward your grounded elbow.

CAUTION: This pose strongly squeezes the abdominal organs and is not recommended for persons with high blood pressure or any type of hernia. Remember, less is more, especially in the beginning. Make a modest twist by sliding your elbow through a belt loop you have placed over your foot and around your knee. If your abdomen cramps, stop doing the pose and go back to Pose 3.

POSE 5. **YOGA LEG LIFTS / URDHVA PRASARITA PADASANA**

There are three possible methods for doing this pose. Choose the one that suits your current abilities, beginning with Version A, as the low back is the most secure in that position.

Version A

➤**1.** Lie on your back with your arms extended to the side and your legs straight out on the floor. ➤**2.** Bring both knees to your chest and then extend them straight up. ➤**3.** Lift the head for additional safety and support, and gaze toward your knees. ➤**4.** Lower one leg until it's 4–10 inches off the floor, and then inhale as you lift it back up. ➤**5.** Exhale to lower the legs, inhale to lift them back up. ➤**6.** Repeat 3 rounds, alternating the legs each round.

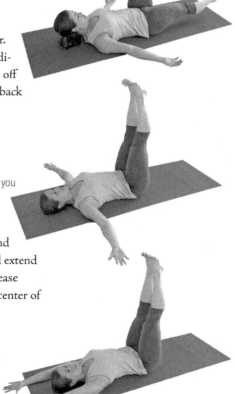

Version B

➤**1.** Repeat steps 1–2 from Version A. ➤**2.** Use one exhale to lower both legs together.

Hint: Control your legs from the center of your clock face, pulling it strongly in and up toward your chest as you exhale. If you feel any strain in your low back, again lift your head and gaze toward your knees.

Version C

➤**1.** Lie on your back with your arms extended overhead, legs straight out on the floor. ➤**2.** Bend your knees to your chest and extend both legs straight up. ➤**3.** Keep your head on the floor and extend from your side waist toward your fingers. ➤**4.** Press the back of your palms into the floor to release tension in the neck. ➤**5.** Exhale and lower the legs as you strongly draw in and up through the center of your clock face. ➤**6.** Repeat for 3–6 rounds.

Hint: When you create full stability of your clock face in this pose, your gluteal muscles will also contract.

CAUTION: When you feel your neck tense, know that the center of your clock face has lifted. This is a clue that you need to develop more awareness and control of the transverse abdominus. Go back to Version A.

POSE 6. **BASIC LYING TWIST / JATHARA PARIVARTANASANA**

The following pose helps tone the diagonal stomach muscles, known as the internal and external obliques.

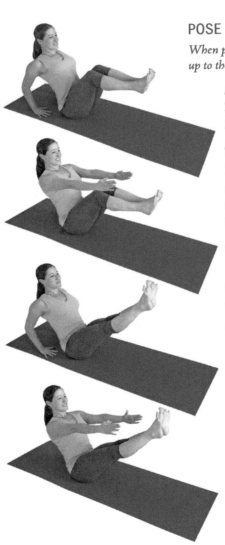

➤**1.** Lie on your back and stretch your arms out to either side to make a 'T' shape, with the palms turned up and the inner shoulders drawn down toward your waist. ➤**2.** Bend your knees in toward your chest. ➤**3.** Keeping the knees closer to your chest than the navel, roll over your hip to twist your knees to the right any amount, stopping 6–10 inches or more from the floor. ➤**4.** Press the back of the right arm down and extend out to the left to keep your shoulder blades in contact with the floor. ➤**5.** As you exhale, drop the lower belly in and turn from the center of your clock face to the left. Bring your left ribs any amount closer to the floor. ➤**6.** Repeat with the knees dropping to the left. ➤**7.** Hold for 3–5 breaths and repeat each side 2–3 times.

Hint: Be certain the knees are closer to your chest than your navel to elongate and release the spine. When you're clearly using your stomach muscles and feel sensations along your spine, be confident that reciprocal inhibition is working for you. These sensations are an indication of tension and spasm leaving your back muscles.

CAUTION: In the beginning, less is more. Complete the twist with the knees as high as 10-12 inches from the floor. As you progress, your body will allow your knees to lower to 6-10 inches off the floor without strain. As always, listen to your body.

POSE 7. **BOAT POSE / PARIPURNA NAVASANA**

When practicing this pose, master Version A with a straight spine before moving forward to Version B. Build up to the most advanced version your body will allow without negative pain or injury.

Hint: To help maintain the lift of your chest and spine, imagine an invisible cord attaching your kidneys to your knees in all versions.

Hint 2: Remember that the feet control the hips, so spread your soles and lift your arches.

Version A

➤**1.** Sit on the floor, legs straight, with your hands 6–8 inches behind you. ➤**2.** Bend your knees and place your feet on the floor. ➤**3.** Inhale and lift your low back and chest so you're sitting on top of your sitting bones, not rolling back onto your sacrum. ➤**4.** Exhale and lift your feet to bring your shins parallel to the floor.

Version B

➤**1.** Repeat steps 1–4 in Version A. ➤**2.** Extend your fingers toward your toes as you draw your shoulders back and down to maintain the lift of the chest. ➤**3.** Compact your outer shins and spread your toes. ➤**4.** Hold for 3–5 breaths.

Version C

➤**1.** Keep your hands on the floor and repeat steps 1–4 in Version A. ➤**2.** Exhale and straighten your legs as much as possible without dropping your chest. ➤**3.** Reach your toes up and out while you compact your legs. ➤**4.** Hold for 3–5 breaths.

Version D

➤**1.** Repeat steps 1–3 from Version C. ➤**2.** Extend your fingers past your knees as you draw your shoulders back and down to maintain the lift of the chest. ➤**3.** Charge the invisible cord connecting your kidneys to your knees. Keep the connection strong. ➤**4.** Drop your shoulders to lift your chest. Reach your toes and crown upward and keep your spine lifted. ➤**5.** Hold for 3–5 breaths.

Alternate Low Back Sequence

Now that you've had time to explore your body practicing the poses in the Basic Low Back, Basic Neck and Shoulder, and Abdominal Toning sequences, you're ready to progress to this Alternate Low Back Sequence. As with any sequence, there may be poses that you really love and others you're not as fond of. Do your best to practice each of the poses in the order presented and observe the areas of your body that experience some relief. As always, listen to your body. If a pose makes your body feel bad after you've tried it three times; then it's time to omit

that pose until something else changes, or until you have an opportunity to speak with an experienced yoga teacher. Sometimes we need to evolve into a pose; again, be patient and do the poses you can.

This sequence contains 19 poses that will initially require 50–60 minutes to complete (you'll complete the poses more quickly as they become more familiar to you). If time is at a premium, you can enjoy a well-balanced but shorter sequence by stopping after Pose 13.

POSE 1. ALTERNATE KNEES TO CHEST /APANASANA

A good beginning for your low back practice, this pose will awaken the transverse abdominus, and also warm, tone, and lengthen the psoas muscles. Refer to Pose 2 in the Abdominal Progressions on page 34.

➤**1.** Draw your right knee toward your armpit and press down and out with the opposite leg. ➤**2.** Keep 3:00 and 9:00 of the clock face level. ➤**3.** Inhale and lift the straight leg up as far as possible. ➤**4.** Exhale and lower the leg 6–10 inches from the floor, holding for 2 breaths. ➤**5.** Repeat each side 3 times.

Inner Action: Pay special attention to pulling the center of your clock face in and up as you lower and reach the straight leg out on your exhalation.

Hint: Remember to turn the straight leg thigh deeply in so the back thigh and knee becomes broad and the knee and toes point up.

POSE 2. ALTERNATING KNEE CURL-UPS /APANASANA VARIATION

This pose more completely warms and tones the psoas muscles, plus it tones the transverse abdominus. It uses resistance to helps us connect to and tone the lower abdominal muscles.

➤**1.** Follow Version B in the Abdominal Progressions Pose 3 on page 34. ➤**2.** Hold onto your right kneecap at arm's length, pressing the knee into your hands, and keep the knee stable and vertical. ➤**3.** Curl the chest up toward the knee one third of the way and gaze straight ahead. ➤**4.** Inhale, as you lift the straight leg up. Exhale, lower the leg to 6-10 inches from the floor and hold for 2 breaths. ➤**5.** Repeat each side 2 or 3 times.

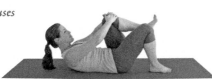
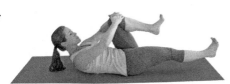

Hint: Be certain to keep the center of the clock face pressing down onto the floor, elbows lifted, and inner shoulders down.

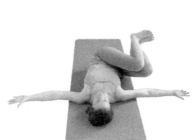

POSE 3. **YOGI CURL-UPS**

Continue to create abdominal tone, including the rectus abdominus, transverse abdominus, internal and external obliques, and the upper psoas muscles with this pose.

➤**1.** Repeat the instructions from the Progressive Abdominal Toning, Pose 1, on page 33.
➤**2.** Hold your elbows in front of your chest, OR cross your arms behind your head as needed to support your neck. ➤**3.** Curl up one third of the way, eyes gazing at your knees. ➤**4.** On the second round, add a twist by bringing the left shoulder toward your right knee, then your right shoulder toward the left knee. ➤**5.** Hold each side for 3–5 breaths and repeat 2–3 times.

Hint: Keep the center of the pelvic clock on the floor. Observe which side in the twist seems weaker, and hold that side longer.

Inner Action: As you exhale and twist, connect the bottom front ribs to the opposite inner groin.

POSE 4. **BASIC LYING TWIST / JATHARA PARIVARTANASANA**

This pose tones the diagonal stomach muscles, the internal and external obliques, as well as the transverse abdominus, and the upper psoas muscles. Refer back to the Abdominal Progressions sheet, Pose 6, page 00 for basic information.

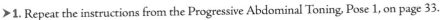

➤**1.** Bend your knees in toward your chest, arms out to the side, palms turned up and inner shoulders drawn down toward your waist. ➤**2.** Keeping the knees well above the navel, roll over your hip to carry your knees to the right, stopping 6–10 inches or greater from the floor. ➤**3.** Press down with the arm on the same side as your knees to turn your chest and belly. ➤**4.** Repeat each side 2–3 times.

Hint 1: In order to unwind your spine with ease, turn your head in the same direction as your knees and gaze toward that hand on the first round. On the second round, turn your head in the opposite direction.

Hint 2: If your spine is particularly stiff, you may place your knees on a block to stay in the pose longer. Add long slow deep breathes to release the diaphragm and open the chest. Continue to ask your belly to turn when you exhale.

Inner Action: Mentally connect and draw from the right groin to the left bottom ribs to turn the upper belly toward the floor.

POSE 5. **SUPINE UPPER BACK TWIST / SUPTA MARICHYASANA III**

The variation of the pose presented here is excellent for removing tension in the upper back, neck, and shoulders, as well as toning all the abdominals. It also lengthens the latissimus dorsi, as well as the mid and upper trapezius. Choose Version A, B, or both from the Progressive Abdominal Toning, Pose 4, on page 34.

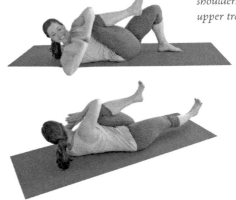

➤**1.** Bend both knees, feet on the floor, and bring one knee in toward your chest. ➤**2.** Capture the knee with the opposite elbow. ➤**3.** Be certain to keep the knee stable, i.e., perpendicular to the floor, as you twist the upper body toward the knee. ➤**4.** Keep the clock face stable. ➤**5.** Hold for 3–5 breaths and repeat each side twice.

Hint: Modify the twist using a belt loop around your knee. {show close up photo again}

Inner Action: Press your palms together as you move the hip of the same side away from your waist to insure that 3:00 and 9:00 stay level. Observe the deeper twist of your belly.

POSES 6, 7, 8. **STRAP STRETCH I, II, III / SUPTA PADANGUSTHASANA SERIES**

This foundational pose series has three leg positions — up, out and over. Up lengthens the low back and hamstrings (shown in Stretch I), out lengthens the inner leg or adductors (Stretch II), and over lengthens the outer leg and side body (Stretch III). Please refer to Poses 3 and 4 of the Basic Low Back Sequence on page 24 for more guidance on Strap Stretch I and III, the up and over positions.

POSE 6. **STRAP STRETCH I–LEG UP**

➤**1.** Place the belt on your right foot and take your right leg up as high as possible without bending your knee. ➤**2.** Press your left inner thigh down and lengthen the leg out through your heel. ➤**3.** When you exhale, extend the right heel toward the ceiling; as you inhale, draw down from the back of your right knee to the floor. ➤**4.** Maintain the balance of your clock face by moving the right hip away from your waist and toward the opposite thigh. ➤**5.** Hold for 5–7 breaths and repeat with the left leg.

Hint: The hamstring muscles offer great resistance. If you tighten your kneecap when stretching the leg that is up, the principle of reciprocal inhibition will confirm that your hamstring is indeed lengthening.

Inner Action: Reach out through both legs as you extend your spine from the center of the clock face out the crown of your head.

POSE 7. **STRAP STRETCH II–LEG OUT TO THE SIDE**

➤**1.** Make a small loop in the belt so a long tail remains. Place the loop around your right foot. ➤**2.** With the right leg straight up, hold the strap in your right hand with a straight arm. ➤**3.** Place the excess strap behind your neck and shoulder. Start with the left elbow bent to hold the belt close to the shoulder. ➤**4.** Place the block outside the right thigh, close to the hip for support. ➤**5.** Turn the right leg out in the socket and draw it up toward your shoulder any amount. ➤**6.** Carry the leg out to the side while attempting to keep the opposite hip on the floor. ➤**7.** Reach the left arm out to pull the belt taught. ➤**8.** Receive the support of the block. Keep the outside of that foot parallel to the floor. ➤**9.** Extend the inner right leg toward the heel as you draw the center of your clock face toward the left. ➤**10.** Hold for 5–7 breaths, up to 1 minute, and then repeat with the other leg.

Hint: Continue to press down and out with your left leg, roll that thigh deep in. Same applies when repeated on other side.

Inner Action: Activate the gluteal muscles in this pose to help keep the opposite hip down on the floor. Draw from the outer right foot and knee in toward the buttock as if to connect your buttocks to your tailbone.

CAUTION: This position is most challenging to your core strength, i.e., the transverse abdominus and gluteal muscles. Therefore use the support of the block to avoid misaligning the pelvis. This will help you keep 3:00 and 9:00 on the horizontal line. Misaligning the pelvis means also misaligning the low back.

POSE 8. **STRAP STRETCH III–LEG ACROSS THE BODY**

➤**1.** Extend the left leg (as shown in the photo) out of the hip and carry it across your body, roll onto the outside of your right hip completely, and rest your foot on the floor or a block. Stack the hips one on top of the other so the clock face is perpendicular to the floor. ➤**2.** Straighten your left leg and spread the toes. ➤**3.** Extend your left arm alongside your head as you move the right hip away from your waist. ➤**4.** Hold for 5–7 breaths, up to 1 minute, and then repeat with the other leg.

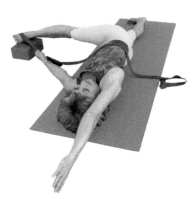

Hint: Be certain to move the top hip away from your waist to balance and decompress your lower back, keeping 3:00 and 9:00 stacked.

Inner Action: Lift the bottom of your belly in and up toward your chest as you press the center top thigh away from your chest to create more length in your spine.

CAUTION: If you have any pinching in the groin of the extended leg, or in the low back or hip, place a block under your foot, as shown in the photograph.

POSE 9. **TRACTION TWIST / SUPTA MATSYANGASANA**

Consider this a first-aid pose: it offers traction for the low back, lengthens the psoas and quadricep muscles, extends the quadratus lumborum and latissimus dorsi, and tones the gluteal muscles.

➤**1.** Place both feet on the floor, wider than your hips. ➤**2.** Drop your knees to the left and align your right knee with your nose. ➤**3.** Extend from your outer right hip toward your knee, allowing your pelvis to lift about halfway up. ➤**4.** Curl the tailbone toward your pubis, and then draw the navel in and up toward your chest. ➤**5.** Hold for 3 breaths. Repeat each side twice.

Hint: Flex your feet to protect your knees. Especially draw the little toe back toward your outer knee.

Inner Action: Extend from your hip to your knee as you draw the center of your clock face in and over to bring your right hip back toward the floor any amount. The same applies when you repeat on other side.

CAUTION: If your right knee suffers any discomfort, please honor that and place a block under the knee to support it both above and below the joint. If any knee pain persists, stop doing the pose.

POSE 10. **PELVIC LIFTS / SETU BANDHA SARVANGASANA**

Stabilize your hips with this pose, which lengthens the quadricep muscles, tones the gluteal muscles, and integrates the psoas muscles on both sides.

➤**1.** Sitting on the floor with knees bent, align your toes with the edge of your mat or an imaginary line, feet hips width apart. ➤**2.** Slide your hips toward your feet so your knees are right over your ankles. ➤**3.** Lie on your back with your arms by your side. ➤**4.** Choose Version A with the block, or Version B with the belt (as described below). ➤**5.** Once the block or belt is in place, curl your tail and slide your knees forward to lift your hips. ➤**6.** Press your heels down to lift your hips higher. ➤**7.** Turn the upper arms under your chest, shoulders blades moving toward the spine. ➤**8.** Press your arms down to raise your breastbone toward your chin in order to elongate your spine and protect your lower back. ➤**9.** Repeat the lift 3 times, holding for 3–5 breaths.

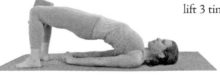

Version A

Begin by holding a block between your knees to tone the inner thighs and release the outer hips and low back as you lift your hips.

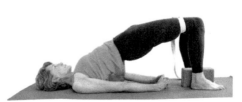

Version B

Place a belt loop approximately 4–6 inches above your knees. Keep your feet hips width apart. As you lift your hips, press out into the belt to activate and tone the gluteal muscles. This version is an excellent choice if you experience low-back or gluteal weakness, or sacroiliac instability.

Hint: To keep your neck in good balance, lift your chin slightly before strongly lifting your chest.

Inner Action: On an exhale, sink your heels and upper arms into the floor, opening the back of your knee to further raise your hips and chest.

CAUTION 1: If this pose causes your low back to pinch, lower your hips 10 even 20 percent and wait for your psoas muscles to release, or choose to place your feet up on a bench or step. Doing so will relieve the pinch and create more length in your lower spine.

CAUTION 2: If you feel any pinching in the inner knee joint, step your feet slightly wider—still use the belt as a guide, but not the block. If the pinching continues, you may also try lifting your feet higher.

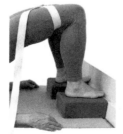

POSE 11. **HALF FISH POSE /ARDHA MATSYASANA**

This pose will help you connect to and tone the back of the neck, mid-trapezius, and rhomboid muscles. See Pose 4 in the Basic Neck and Shoulders Sequence, page 00, for full details.

➤**1.** Lie on your back with your knees partially bent. ➤**2.** Bend your elbows and place them 8–10 inches away from your ribs. ➤**3.** Turn your upper arms completely out so the shoulder blades lie flat between your chest and the floor. ➤**4.** Lift your chin until the back of your crown is in contact with the floor. ➤**5.** Press the back of your head and elbows down to lift your chest up. ➤**6.** Balance equally on your elbows and the back of your crown. ➤**7.** Hold the pose until your shoulders, neck, and arms become mildly fatigued—about 3–5 breaths. Repeat.

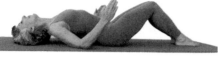

Hint: Press the elbows diagonally down into the floor to draw the inner shoulder blades down away from the neck and spread them apart.

Inner Action: With your inhale, send the breath into your legs and your chest simultaneously. Draw your organs in and up from the center of your clock face to your chest.

POSE 12. **SUPINE BOUND ANGLE ROCK / SUPTA BADDHA KONASANA VARIATION**

This pose gently balances the pelvis, stabilizing the sacroiliac and hip joints.

➤**1.** Lie on your back. Join the soles of your feet and hold your ankles. ➤**2.** Draw your feet toward your chest and keep your knees wide apart, as if they're held open with a pole. ➤**3.** Rock slowly side to side over the crest of your hips. ➤**4.** Allow your head to follow as you reach each knee to touch the floor. Repeat 2–3 times.

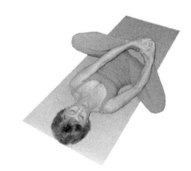

Hint: If you can't reach your feet or ankles with your hands, use a belt to capture your feet and draw them toward your chest.

Inner Action: Notice any sore or uneven spots along the crest of your hips. Pause on them and add your smooth, deep breaths to encourage them to melt away.

POSE 13. **DOWNWARD FACING DOG / ADHO MUKHA SVANASANA**

This pose provides good extension of the muscles of the arms and legs, which creates length and space in the spine by applying a fundamental principle of alignment, i.e., the legs extend the spine. For detailed reminders, please refer to Pose 6 of the Basic Neck and Shoulder Sequence, page 30.

Version B—hands on the floor

➤**1.** From a kneeling position, place the palms ahead of your shoulders, with the middle fingers running parallel to each other. ➤**2.** As usual, press your hands down to lift your hips into the air. ➤**3.** Move your pubic bone back between your legs to lift your hips further up. ➤**4.** Press the inner palms and index knuckles down to extend up your inner arms. ➤**5.** Deepen the crease at the top of your thigh. ➤**6.** Wrap your outer armpit toward the floor as you lift the inner arm up. ➤**7.** Keep your heels lifted as you straighten your legs as much as possible. ➤**8.** Relax your neck. Hold the pose for 5–7 breaths.

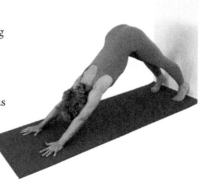

Hint: If you have very short hamstrings, you'll need to keep your knees bent. Spinal extension is the priority.

Inner Action: As you extend the palm of the hand forward, continue to press your mid-thigh back to contain the belly and lengthen more fully the front of the spine.

CAUTION: As always choose the version of the pose that is right for you. If you feel any discomfort in your low back, better to choose Version A with your hands on a wall or ledge (described on page 30).

POSE 14. **LUNGES / VANARASANA**

Long hours spent sitting shorten the muscles of the front thigh and groin, limiting the movement of our legs and spine. In order to warm the muscles of the front thigh and achieve good extension, please practice the lunge in the three ways shown to fully lengthen the quadriceps and psoas muscles.

Version A—Low Lunge
(see Pose 5 of the Basic Low Back Sequence, page 25)

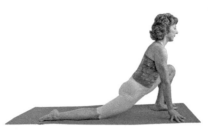

➤**1.** Begin kneeling on all fours. ➤**2.** Swing your left foot forward and place your ankle under your knee. ➤**3.** With your right knee down, slide the right knee back until you feel a good stretch on that front thigh. ➤**4.** Align the front knee with its own hip by turning the knee out. ➤**5.** Balance and flatten the front of your clock face. ➤**6.** Hold for 3–5 breaths. Change sides, and then repeat.

Inner Action: On an exhalation, draw the center of your clock face in and up as you reach down and back with the rear knee.

CAUTION: Avoid excess pressure on your knee by placing a blanket under your knee and full length of your shin. Also, place blocks under your hands to keep from collapsing the "tube" of your front spine as shown. Use the blocks as high as needed.

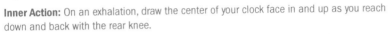

Version B—Low Lunge, Hands on knee
(see Pose 7 of the Basic Neck & Shoulder Sequence, page 31)

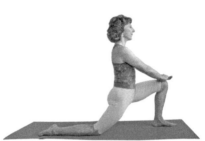

➤**1.** Repeat steps 1–4 in Low Lunge, Version A. ➤**2.** Ground down through the left heel to lift your clock face in and up. ➤**3.** Raise your hands up onto your left knee. ➤**4.** Balance your clock face. ➤**5.** Hold for 3–5 breaths. Change sides, and then repeat.

Inner Action: As you exhale, sink the front heel into the floor to press your tail forward and lift the bottom of your belly.

Version C—High Lunge

➤**1.** Repeat steps 1–4 in Version A, and then lift your right knee up to straighten the leg behind you. ➤**2.** Make your right foot as vertical to the floor as possible. ➤**3.** Press the ball of the right foot down as you lift the ankle up to lift the shin, straighten the knee and float the thigh. ➤**4.** Lift the outer right hip so 3:00 and 9:00 remain parallel to the floor. ➤**5.** Extend the inner rear leg back as the inner front knee extends forward. ➤**6.** Reach the breastbone forward, with the neck in a neutral position. ➤**7.** Hold for 3–5 breaths and change sides. Repeat again on both sides.

Hint: Turn the front knee out to squeeze that hip in toward your tailbone, clearly aligning the center of your hip and knee, thus maintaining the parallel railroad tracks of the legs and pelvis; this will stabilize your hips, further balance 3:00 and 9:00, and keep your low back extending evenly.

Inner Action: Draw the center of the clock face in and up toward your chest equal to the extension back of the inner rear leg. Lift your collarbones to elongate your chest, with the neck in a neutral position.

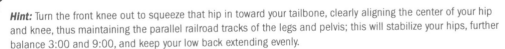

POSE 15. **DOWNWARD FACING DOG / ADHO MUKHA SVANASANA**

As physics plays a roll in yoga, this variation of dog pose—done by placing the feet on blocks at the wall—offers added relief for the low back. Practicing this way effectively decompresses the lumbar spine, allowing the "tube" of the spine to open. Please refer to Pose 6 of the Basic Neck and Shoulder Sequence on page 30 for a full description of Versions A and B.

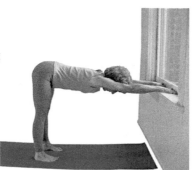

Version C—Feet on blocks at the wall

➤**1.** Place the blocks on the lowest level hip-width apart against the wall. ➤**2.** Start on your hands and knees, with your feet close to the blocks; then walk your hands 6 inches forward of your shoulders. ➤**3.** As usual, press your hands down to lift your hips into the air. ➤**4.** Place one foot at a time on a block with your toes reaching off the edge and your heels touching the wall, with the foot at a 45-degree angle. ➤**5.** Press the inner palms down to extend up your inner arms to your hips. ➤**6.** Then roll the skin of the back leg over your buttocks to extend the back of your legs and spine. ➤**7.** Anchoring your heels to the wall, slowly straighten your legs as much as possible. ➤**8.** As your heels press into the wall, lift up from your mid-calf to your buttocks. ➤**9.** Relax your neck. Hold the pose for 5–7 breaths.

Hint: If you have very short hamstrings, you'll need to keep your knees bent. Spinal extension is the priority.

Inner Action: As you roll the skin from the bottom of the buttock into your lumbar spine, resist and lift your forearms away from the floor to maintain the extension of your spine.

CAUTION: If your spine is tender, choose the option of dog pose with your hands on the wall on ledge.

POSE 16. **STANDING CHAIR TWIST / MARICHYASANA III VARIATION**

This pose relieves tension along the spine by stretching the very small muscles that connect one vertebra to another. It also builds tone in the legs to help you gain length in your spine.

Twisting poses are necessary yet challenging for the spine, as it's difficult to maintain length while you twist. This pose is engineered to maintain the length and space in your spine while you twist. You may also refer to Twisting Progressions, page 63, for other twisting postures.

➤**1.** Begin by placing a chair against the wall with a block on the seat. Please note that there is no mat under the chair, which is braced against the wall. ➤**2.** Stand to the side and close to the chair, with your heels elevated on a rolled-up mat. ➤**3.** Place the foot that is closest to the wall on the block: in this photo, the left leg. ➤**4.** Stand in the back of your right leg by aligning the center of your hip with your knee and ankle. ➤**5.** Lift your chest and spine from the center of your clock face and roll your shoulders back. ➤**6.** With your right hand, hold the left knee to keep it stationary; place your left hand on the wall behind your left shoulder. ➤**7.** Imagine a line from your right inner ankle to the crown of your head, aligning the center of each of the 4 diaphragms. ➤**8.** Inhale. As you exhale, twist toward the wall, turning from the bottom of your belly. Keep your left knee stationary as you turn. ➤**9.** Turn your spine around your center line. With each exhale, empty your belly and continue to twist your spine incrementally from the bottom to the top. ➤**10.** Hold for 3–5 breaths. Repeat each side twice.

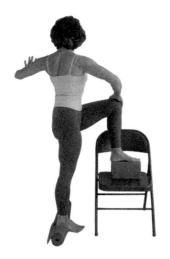

Hint: Avoid leaning forward onto the top of your right thigh. Pull the top thigh back by micro-bending your right knee; in other words, keep the tube of your leg evenly balanced.

Inner Action: Lower your left hip to balance 3:00 and 9:00 as you lift your left ribs up and turn any amount more.

Note: both the Hint and Inner Action applies to both sides.

POSE 17. STANDING HAND-TO-FOOT POSE / UTTHITA HASTA PADANGUSTHASANA

Now that you're warmed up from the previous 16 poses, you're ready for this more challenging pose. It lengthens the hamstrings, extends and decompresses the spine, and makes your legs strong.

➤**1.** Place the chair at the wall for stability and stand back one leg length. ➤**2.** Stand Erect as shown in Pose 7 in the Basic Low Back Sequence on page 25. ➤**3.** Place one foot up on the chair back.* ➤**4.** Micro-bend your standing knee, as in the previous pose, to vertically align your standing leg: ankle, knee, and hip to shoulder. ➤**5.** Straighten your top leg completely. ➤**6.** Lengthen from the back of both knees toward your hips to draw 6:00 back to the center of your pelvic floor and extend the back of your legs. ➤**7.** Now lift from the pelvic floor and the bottom of your belly up through your chest to the crown of your head. ➤**8.** Raise your arms and lift your palms upward out of your hips to lengthen your spine. ➤**9.** Do your best to level your clock face so your hipbones are parallel to the floor. ➤**10.** Hold the pose 5–7 breaths with each leg.

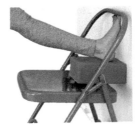

Hint: In order to make the pose match the current length of your hamstrings, you may need to place your foot on the seat of the chair, or on a block on the chair. The block has three heights to choose from: low, medium, and tall. Remember, the spine must extend completely, so less is more.

Inner Action: As you reach into your heels, lift the invisible line from the inside tip of your tailbone, along your front spine, through your soft pallet, to the crown of your head.

CAUTION: If you find balance to be a challenge, place the chair sideways against a wall before placing your foot on the chair.

POSE 18. UPWARD FACING DOG POSE / URDHVA MUKHA SVANASANA

In this pose, you'll extend the front spine and tone the spinal muscles to help build the stability of your lower back; the bolster and the blocks minimize joint compression.

Version A

Lie on a lengthwise bolster with the middle of your abdomen in contact with the front edge, knees supported.

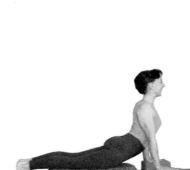

➤**1.** Place your hands close to your hips with blocks under each hand. ➤**2.** Curl your toes and firm your thighs by pressing your pelvis down and your thighs up. ➤**3.** Roll your shoulders back, and then press the bottom of your breast bone forward. ➤**4.** Extend your legs back and expand your chest forward before lifting. ➤**5.** Inhale, curl your chest up, and straighten your arms as much as possible. ➤**6.** Exhale and lower your chest back down. ➤**7.** Repeat 4–5 times; then lift and hold for 3 breaths.

Hint: Continue to lengthen your spine by reaching back with your legs and forward with your chest.

CAUTION: Go only as high as possible without negative pain in your low back. You control this by how much you straighten your arms.

POSE 19. **INVERTED LAKE / VIPARITA KARANI**

You've earned it! Now is the time to rest and relax your spine, legs, and mind, while improving your circulation and boosting your confidence.

At the end of each practice sequence, it's important to rest in order to integrate the new muscle memory and restore our nervous system. This pose is guaranteed to do just that.

➤**1.** Fold several blankets 8–10 inches in width until you have a stack 6–8 inches tall, or use a standard yoga bolster. ➤**2.** Place the blanket stack or the bolster 6–8 inches away from the wall and sit next to it with your back and hips touching the wall. ➤**3.** Swing your legs to the side and place one shoulder in position on the floor. ➤**4.** Roll over onto your back so your hips end up on the blanket stack or bolster. ➤**5.** Place your arms either straight out to the sides at shoulder height, palms up, or in cactus pose, as shown in the photo. ➤**6.** Remain in this position 7–10 minutes. ➤**7.** To come out, bend your knees to slide your hips down onto the floor. ➤**8.** Draw your knees into your chest and roll to your right side.

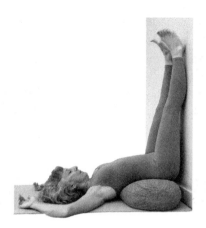

Hint: More important than touching your legs to the wall is feeling the support under your lower back ribs, so adjust the position of the bolster by lifting your hips and pulling it up under your back ribs until your kidneys are supported. Make the belly soft and neutral. Then completely let go and relax.

CAUTION: If you feel any pinching in your lower back, you may either have your hips too close to the wall for the length of your hamstrings, or the bolster has been pulled up too high under your back, resulting in the pelvis losing support. Experiment and adjust.

Elements for Successful Relaxation

There are different approaches to relaxation currently offered in the health care field. Some of you may have experienced one or several of them; however, I'll review them again here in order to help clearly identify them so you can choose which one works best for you.

In *progressive relaxation*, you inhale, squeeze the muscle or body part tight, and then let go completely on the exhale. With this approach, you can work your way progressively through the body, beginning either with the feet or the face and head.

In *autogenic / progressive relaxation* training, you imagine your body parts getting warm, and then warm and heavy, using your imagination, rather than muscle movement.

In *yogic relaxation* practice, you use both imagination and the breath, as well as body position, to create a deep sense of stillness and a conscious letting go.

There are several elements to setting up a positive yogic relaxation practice.

Choose a yoga posture that will assist your muscular and physiological relaxation. There are three versions of supported Corpse Pose / Savasana to choose from in this book: "Suspended Relaxation" (Basic Low Back Sequence, page 278), "Calves on a Chair Seat" (Basic Low Back Sequence, page 27), and "Over a Horizontal Blanket" (Basic Neck and Shoulder Sequence, page 32).

Two of my favorite poses for personal use and as a foundation for my therapeutic yoga classes are the Inverted Lake Pose / Viparita Karani, in which the hips are placed on a blanket stack or bolster and the legs rest on the wall, and Supported Pelvic Lift / Setu Bandha Sarvangasana, in which the shoulders drop back and the body is fully supported, with the legs resting straight at the same height as the hips. Both these poses can be found in the Six Basic Restorative Poses on page 47. The benefits of each of these poses can be found on the pages mentioned.

Choose the best environment. Research shows that if the lights are dim and our bodies are warm, we're more likely to relax. Choose a space where you can be quiet and undisturbed. Dim the lights and cover yourself with a blanket, including your hands and feet.

Adjust your Breath. Once you're comfortable and warm, begin to make your exhalation longer than your inhalation. Start small and continue to lengthen your exhale so it approaches half the length of your inhale to access the parasympathetic system and reverse the stress response.

Add Mental Awareness. Beginning at your feet, progressively relax one part of your body at a time. Inhale your breath into each body part to connect your mind more fully to your body; as you exhale, let go completely.

Follow a Theme. There are many themes you can employ that will deepen your relaxation practice. Certainly the breath is the most important and pivotal key; in addition, the mind can be directed in a variety of different ways. I offer you three possibilities that may be helpful.

1. Consider your physiology: With your exhalations, give your attention to letting go of the muscles, bones, organs, nerves, and blood vessels, allowing yourself to sink deeper within.

2. Consider your five senses: With your exhalations, give attention to relaxing your jaw and tongue, the bridge of your nose and sinuses, the eyes in their sockets. As you exhale, guide your ears to soften inward; also soften your skin and allow it to spread.

3. Employ visualizations: Use the five elements to create a sense of connection and ease, repeating the visualization of your choice to each part of your body connected to an exhalation. Try one of these, or find another that feels right to you.

   + "I surrender my _____ (body part) to the earth."
   + "I allow my breath to be like water, washing tension away."
   + "I surrender to the space around my body, knowing I am safe."
   + "I feel my body melting like _____ on a warm summer day."

Thoughts for yoga teachers. When guiding a class of students in relaxation, consider the following:

1. Keep the Rhythm of your voice smooth and methodical. Breath deeply so as not to rush your words. Remember: the cranial sacral rhythm is the slowest in the body. The pulse is 3 beats in and 3 beats out—very slow. Match the rhythm of your voice to that.

2. Repeat key Sounds, Words, or Phrases throughout your guided relaxation. For instance, tell your students, "As you exhale, relax your arms, and completely let go." Repeat, "Completely let go."

Six Basic Restorative Poses

Recognizing that stress of any kind can aggravate low back conditions because we tend to hold our breath when we're feeling stressed, it's important that we take the time to unwind and relax to assist the healing process. Refer to the Anatomy of the Low Back on page 22 to review the origin and insertion of the diaphragm.

In this section, I describe six basic restorative poses and some of their benefits. Four of these poses are suitable to hold for long periods of time in order to practice the Essential Elements of Relaxation. Suggested timings will be mentioned in the description for each.

POSE 1. RECLINED BOUND ANGLE POSE / SUPTA BADDHA KONASANA

This pose promotes stability and balance in the pelvis, and broadens the lower abdomen, thus releasing tension and improving circulation to the lower abdominal organs. It also releases tension across the front of the sacrum and lumbar spine, and elevates the chest to sooth the heart and relieve depression. Practice this pose for 7–15 minutes with support under the legs and chest.

➤**1.** Begin by gathering your props: 1 strap, 2 blocks or 2 Three-Minute Eggs, 1 bolster with 1 blanket or 3 blankets. ➤**2.** Place the bolster lengthwise on your mat, with a blanket folded in half or in thirds to go under your head like a pillow. If you don't have a bolster, fold the other two blankets and stack them in place of the bolster, as described in Pranayama Guidelines on page 51. ➤**3.** Sit on the floor, a hand-width away from the bolster or blanket stack. ➤**4.** Make a large loop in the belt, place it over your head, and drop it down to your hips. ➤**5.** Draw the soles of your feet together and toward your groin. ➤**6.** Slide the belt down to cross around the middle of the pelvis, pass over the inside of your legs, and then loop around the outside of your feet. ➤**7.** Slowly draw the belt tighter until the legs are held fast in position, 6-10" away from your groin. ➤**8.** Place the eggs or blocks under your thighs so they offer support, minimizing the stretch on the inner groin. ➤**9.** Lean back on your hands, raise your hips up, and move the flesh of your buttocks toward your feet; then place your hips back down. ➤**10.** Slowly lie back so your chest and ribs are fully supported by the bolster. ➤**11.** Slide the third blanket under your head, checking to see that your forehead is slightly higher than your chin. ➤**12.** Roll your shoulders back, turn your palms up, and relax. ➤**13.** In the beginning, hold this pose for 7–10 minutes. As you become more familiar with the practice, you can hold for as long as 15 minutes. ➤**14.** When you're ready to come out of the pose, lift your knees up and slowly release the strap. ➤**15.** Extend your legs out straight, flex your feet, and tighten your knees; then let go and rest your legs for 1 more minute.

Hint: Slide the belt low down on the back of your hips so it will end up creating traction for your low back. Also, place the buckle of the belt in a location other than on a muscle.

Inner Action: Breath long and deep into your pelvis. Imagine the four corners of your pelvis spreading outward to the four directions. Let go of all tension with your exhalation.

CAUTION: Be sure to tuck your tailbone toward your feet so your lower belly relaxes and drops in. Think of flattening your clock face. If this is difficult to do, or if you have any pinching in your low back, bring your spine closer to the floor by using 2 blankets, or even 1 and ½ blankets under your spine, rather than a bolster.

POSE 2. **SUPPORTED PELVIC LIFT / SETU BANDHA SARVANGASANA, FULLY SUPPORTED**

With the head and neck positioned below the heart, this pose is a mild inversion and offers all the benefits of an inversion. The blood flows into the head to nourish the brain; endorphins are released by changing the pressure on the carotid artery; the organs are extended, relieving pressure on the diaphragm; the chest opens, allowing the heart to pump freely; and the thyroid, parathyroid, thymus, and adrenals are invigorated. This position is an excellent pose to do almost anytime, providing us with deep rest and restoration in a few short minutes! Time in the pose can vary, although 10–15 minutes is recommended. Shorter or longer timings are also possible as noted in the instructions.

➤**1.** Begin with 2 bolsters placed end-to-end, or 4 blankets folded and stacked into two piles, placed end-to-end. ➤**2.** In order to relax your legs completely, place a belt around your calves, as shown in the photo, or around your mid thighs. ➤**3.** Sit with your hips on the bolster and knees bent. ➤**4.** Again lift your hips and move the flesh of your buttocks toward your feet. ➤**5.** Lie back on the bolster with the bottom edge of your shoulder blades hanging on the edge of the bolster. ➤**6.** Your shoulders will not be touching the floor, however, the back of your neck will feel long. ➤**7.** Relax your arms out to the sides. ➤**8.** Hold this position a minimum of 7 minutes or as long as 30 minutes. ➤**9.** To come out, bend your knees and roll to your side. ➤**10.** Rest on your side for 5–10 breaths, and then slowly push yourself up to sitting.

Hint: Hook the bottom tip of your shoulder blades on the edge of the bolster. Fasten them there to roll your top chest down toward the floor.

Inner Action: Take long, slow, deep breaths to experience the expansion of your chest and ribs. Breathe into your top chest as best you can, and let go completely on the exhalation.

CAUTION: If your shoulders are too far off the edge of the bolster, you may experience too much bend in your low back, along with some discomfort. To remedy this, simply slide back up onto the bolster so your top chest is supported, as if you were doing Pose 4, Half Fish Pose, from the Basic Neck and Shoulder Sequence on page 29.

POSE 3. **PRONE TWIST ON A BOLSTER / PRONE BHARADVAJASANA**

Remember this is a first-aid pose for the lumbar spine because it creates space for a herniated disc to be drawn off the nerve and oftentimes moved back into place. This is also a useful pose if you have low-back inflammation as it decompresses your lower spine. In addition, the pose rests and nourishes your organs, which are toned when squeezed.

➤**1.** Sit on the floor with your legs folded to one side and your knees separated. ➤**2.** Place the bolster lengthwise 4–6 inches away from the side of your hip. ➤**3.** Lift your spine from the bottom of your belly. ➤**4.** Exhale to twist your ribs, and then place your chest evenly on the bolster. ➤**5.** Begin by facing your nose in the same direction as your knees; turning your head to the opposite side, as in the photo, is optional. ➤**6.** Hold each side for 1–3 minutes, breathing evenly.

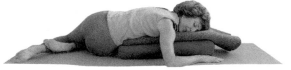

Hint: If you feel any pinching in the lower side of your waist, tuck the flesh of your side buttock under you and away from the bolster to relieve the "kink in the tube."

Inner Action: Breathe into the spaces between your shoulder blades, as well as your lower back.

POSE 4. SLEEPING FROG PRONE ON A BOLSTER

After performing both sides of the Prone Twist on the Bolster, move into this pose to lengthen, release, and return your lower back to its natural curve. Sleeping Frog also compresses the center of your clock face, which softens the lower abdominal organs, supports the low back, and stimulates the reproductive organs to increase vitality.

➤**1.** Place the bolster vertically on the mat. Lie down so that the edge of the bolster makes contact with the center of your clock face. ➤**2.** Drop your knees to the sides of the bolster. ➤**3.** Rest your chest on the floor. ➤**4.** Turn your head one way for approximately 30 seconds, and then the other. ➤**5.** Hold the pose for 1–2 minutes. ➤**6.** Slowly push yourself back to sitting.

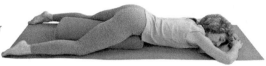

Hint: Position is everything: the edge of the bolster should be no higher than 2–3 inches above your pubic bone. Keep adjusting your position until you find the "sweet spot" where your spine feels completely released.

POSE 5. INVERTED LAKE POSE / VIPARITA KARANI

The benefits of the Inverted Lake Pose match the points given in Pose 2, Supported Pelvic Lift above, with a few modifications. In this pose, the vascular system is also toned as the heart now is asked to pump the blood to the feet against gravity, improving circulation. (See Pose 19 in Alternate Low Back Sequence on page 45 for more details.)

➤**1.** Create your stack of blankets, or use a standard yoga bolster. ➤**2.** Place the bolster 6–8 inches away from the wall. ➤**3.** Sit close to the wall and swing your legs up into position.* ➤**4.** Roll your shoulders back and tuck them in sideways under your chest to relieve any pressure in your neck and throat. ➤**5.** Relax in this position for 7, 10, or 15 minutes. ➤**6.** To come out, bend your knees to slide your hips down onto the floor. ➤**7.** Draw your knees into your chest and roll to your right side.

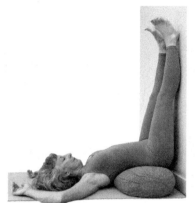

Hint: More important than touching your legs to the wall is feeling the support under your lower back ribs, so adjust the position of the bolster by lifting your hips and pulling it up under your back ribs until your kidneys are supported. Make the belly soft and neutral. Then completely let go and relax.

Note*: If you have difficulty rolling into this position, try this: while lying flat on your back, slide your hips into position and then lift them up to slip the bolster into place.

POSE 6. CORPSE POSE / SAVASANA

As first described in the Basic Low Back Sequence, Pose 13, on page 27, Corpse Pose, Version A is recommended here. The benefits of Suspended Relaxation (Version A) are the softening of the hip joints and low back, the support of the chest offering ease in breathing, and the feeling of lightness through the entire spine.

Version A

➤**1.** Fold one blanket in half lengthwise, place the narrow edge at the back of your waist, and then lie down so your rib cage is lifted. ➤**2.** Place a second blanket under your head with the back of your neck supported. ➤**3.** Elevate your lower legs, with the calves resting on a bolster, knees bent and turned out. ➤**4.** Use your hands to lift your buttocks and move the flesh toward your feet so your lower back lengthens and your hips rest evenly on the floor. ➤**5.** Turn your palms up and draw your inner shoulder blades away from your ears. ➤**6.** Relax in this position for 5–15 minutes, breathing easy. ➤**7.** To come out of the pose, bring your knees together and roll to your right side.

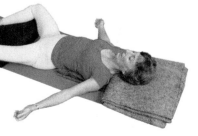

Hint: Check to see that your forehead is slightly higher than your chin; if necessary, fold the blanket for the pillow in halves or thirds for more height.

Yogic Breathing Practice: Pranayama *Guidelines*

Everyone knows how to breathe, right? Seemingly so; however, all too often people find themselves in a shallow breathing pattern. As I mentioned earlier, the more shallow we breath and the more tense our breath, the higher our stress levels can become. When we find ourselves in pain, whether physical, mental, or emotional, our breath becomes constricted. The goal of yoga is to help us learn to reset our rhythm, reduce our stress, and connect with the wisdom of our inner being and body through deep intentional breathing. I recommend you approach this practice as an integral part of your healing journey.

We'll begin with deep breathing while we're lying down, a sensible way to learn some of the basics of *pranayama*, a discipline that will continue to develop and deepen through steady practice. Starting in a supine position removes the effort needed to sit up straight, which means we can breath with ease to help release tension and stress.

There are two primary areas of the body that we need to open when we practice *pranayama*:

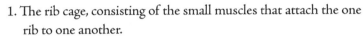
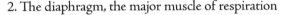

1. The rib cage, consisting of the small muscles that attach the one rib to one another.
2. The diaphragm, the major muscle of respiration

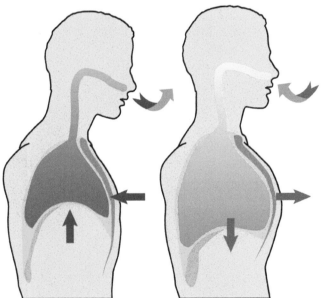

The diaphragm is considered the muscle that separates the conscious mind from the sub-conscious, and thus holds as tension all our unresolved emotions. When we practice deep intentional breathing, we're often able to release the tension, even if we haven't fully "processed" the emotional content. The breathing practice presented here begins with deep relaxation; when emotional or mental content does arise it will tend to disturb our relaxation. I recommend you find a way to process the disturbance by either journaling your in-the-moment concerns before you begin your *pranayama* practice, or you could imagine those thoughts or feelings being placed in a paper bag to be picked up again at the end of your practice. Use any favorite technique you have for clearing yourself, and then begin. In my experience, if the content does need some attending to, it will return to us in our meditation at the end of the practice. The hope is that more clarity will be available to us at that time.

Begin Your Practice

Pranayama, is best done first thing in the morning before our day starts. In the morning our minds tend to be clearer after a night's rest and our body is more relaxed. Set your blankets up the night before and have a timer nearby. Set your alarm 20 minutes earlier to accommodate your practice, complete your morning bathroom cleansing activities, and be sure to drink a glass of water before beginning.

Follow the guidelines below on how to create your set-up, along with the recommended procedure. Add a short meditation at the end of your breathing practice if you like, and then start your day. If your schedule determines that you need to practice asana in the morning before breakfast, then practice *pranayama* before dinner.

Signs of Wrong Practice

Be sure to make your breath relaxed and smooth. If you're grasping, gripping, or gasping for air, you're overdoing. Please let up until you experience smooth, relaxed, deep breathing. Headaches, light-headedness, depression, anxiety, or irritability are signs of tension, or an overly aggressive practice.

If you fall asleep in the beginning, it's not a sign of wrong practice. When sleep overtakes us during *pranayama*, it's an indication that we're indeed expanding our breath capacity, which results in increased levels of CO_2. This can trigger the automatic sleep response, which brings us back to normal breathing. As our practice develops, our capacity to hold higher CO_2 levels increases, as does the carefree bliss we experience through this practice.

Philosophy

On the inhalation, invite peace, light, and beauty to enter your body with the breath. Soften your skin to receive what cannot be controlled and let yourself feel the sensation of space in and around your body. On the exhalation, release distress or tension back to the Source within you for transformation.

Blanket Folding for Pranayama

Choose two dense wool or cotton blankets; fiberfill and polyester blankets slip and slide, offering no real support or security for our chest and spine. Follow the folding instructions below.

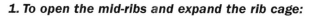

You can practice *pranayama* using either of these approaches; try them both to experience their different benefits.

1. To open the mid-ribs and expand the rib cage:

Use one blanket folded in half lengthwise. Lie on it horizontally across your mid back. Slide your head and shoulders over and off the blanket, allowing your bottom shoulder tips to remain on the blanket so your top chest opens. Refer to Pose 13, Basic Neck and Shoulder Sequence on page 32.

2. To open the diaphragm:

Fold two blankets lengthwise down the center, with the wide folds edge to edge. Then stack the blankets with the center folds on opposite sides of the stack; keep all the edges even to create a stable base. Use a third blanket folded in half, thirds or fourths as a pillow. Refer to Pose 13, Basic Low Back Sequence, on page 27.

Placing your body on the stacked blankets:

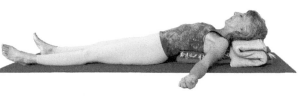

Sit one-hand's distance away from the blanket stack and carefully place and center your hips on the floor. Lie back onto the blankets, with your spine in the middle. Slide the third blanket under your head. In proper head position, the chin is slightly lower than the forehead. Extend your legs out straight, and then allow them to relax and fall open. Turn the upper arms back to draw the inner shoulder blades away from your ears and create a feeling of openness in your top chest as you did in version 1 with the horizontal blanket.

Hint: Check that the bottom front ribs are higher than your hip bones and that the bridge of the nose is higher than the breastbone.

CAUTION: If you feel a pinch in your low back either lift your hips with your hands and slide the buttock flesh toward your feet, or lower the stack of blankets one layer at a time until you find relief.

Pranayama *Practice Guidelines*

Hint: Try adding the sound of "Hum" on the inhalation and "Sa" on the exhalation; these sounds create what is named the *Ujjayi breath.* The sounds will help keep your mind from wandering and decrease the likelihood of you falling to sleep. The sounds help to focus the mind in the moment and should only be audible to you.

1. Lie down in either of the versions described above. First RELAX for 5 minutes, become sensitive to any areas in the body where you're holding tension, and consciously let go.
2. Begin by making your exhalation longer than your inhalation; i.e., inhale for 4–6 counts, then exhale for 6–8 counts, and continue this rhythm for 2–3 minutes to awaken your parasympathetic system.
3. Now, imagine your breath becoming wide and then deep on each inhale, without creating any tension in your body, especially in your back, belly, neck, shoulders, and face. Then match the length of your inhale to your exhale, with a slight pause at the top of the inhale, and again at the bottom of the exhale. Continue in this way for 3–5 minutes.

Benefit: Notice the deep sense of calm that arises from this simple practice. You could stop the practice here by simply returning to normal breathing and relaxation for 5 minutes, or continue to items a–d in the next section.

Deepening the Practice

To more completely release tension in your diaphragm, low back or ribs, continue to deepen your practice by adding the following elements. You'll need to extend your inhalation to be longer than your exhalation, but without causing any tension. In this way, you'll cultivate an increased lung capacity and the sense of bliss mentioned earlier. As this part of the *pranayama* practice is more rigorous in mental focus and more stimulating to your central nervous system, continue to practice this section for only 5 minutes.

a. Pay attention to the inner action of the breath. Guide the sensation of the inhale from the opening of your nostrils, to the back of your throat, down the back of your spine, and into your pelvis and legs. The breath will become obviously cyclical, as there will be sensations of the breath, both descending deep into the body, while simultaneously rising up into the chest. This direction will bring your mind into contact with your inner body and help you stay grounded and relaxed. Alternate this breath awareness with the fully expanded chest breath discussed next.

b. Further lengthen your inhale. Begin by exhaling completely, and then inhale down your back body as in part 'a.' Imagine the sensation of the breath being like water running down the sides of a glass and filling it from the bottom to the top. Expand your bottom ribs into a wide oval to spread and open your diaphragm like the wings of a bird. As your breath transitions from horizontal to vertical, draw the skin of your pubis up to lift the breath up the central channel to touch under your heart. (This is a similar yet more subtle action then when you lift the bottom of your belly.) Pause at the top of your inhale before any gripping begins, and circularly expand your top chest, letting go of all tension in your face and throat.

c. Exhale in a slow, smooth manner. Because your inhale is likely to be longer than your exhale, you may run out of breath before the end of your exhale. If that happens, simply pause and take a small inhale, and then finish the exhale. Be certain to keep your breath smooth. Return to the breath awareness mentioned in 'a' above, relax, let go of any inner tension, and then expand your breath again, repeating parts 'b' and 'c.'

d. Finish the practice by letting the exhale be longer than the inhale for 2–3 minutes. Roll to your right side and relax there, or lie flat on your back with a small blanket fold for a pillow in Corpse Pose for 3–5 minutes. Choose to meditate at this time, or move on with your day.

This entire practice will take approximately 20 minutes.

Self-Applied Back Care Quick Review: Part 1

1. *Name the common causes of back pain.* Most back pain is caused by muscular contraction due to stress or overuse, weak muscles that do not support the back, or is the result of an accident or injury.

2. *When a person with back pain begins a yoga practice, what is the appropriate primary focus?* Remember that gravity creates compression; therefore, if back pain is present, always create length and space in the joints before you begin to strengthen muscles.

3. *What is the key characteristic of a muscle spasm?* A muscle in spasm *tends to remain in spasm* until *acted on by an outside force,* meaning an appropriate yoga pose done in a balanced way with good alignment.

4. *What are the two phases of back pain? Phase 1* is acute pain; *Phase 2* is a weak back with no pain. The pattern repeats until the pain becomes chronic, with the painful days lasting longer and longer.

5. *What is reciprocal inhibition and how can it inform our practice?* Every muscle has an opposite or antagonistic muscle. By contracting one muscle, its opposite muscle will release and lengthen, satisfying the goal of releasing muscle spasms and pain, as well as creating length. The sensation of stretching felt in a muscle can be known to be effective, if and when its opposite muscle is contracting; otherwise the muscle will be holding rather than releasing and lengthening.

6. *What is the cellular structure of scar tissue?* How long does it remain pliable? How does scar tissue affect mobility? Scar tissue forms a chaotic patchwork of fibers, creating an internal band-aid. It will remain pliable for 6–9 months, and then it will become more solid and stronger than the surrounding tissue. Scar tissue does not stretch very well once it's fully formed, thus limiting mobility.

7. *Name the four curves of the spine.* These are the cervical curve, the thoracic curve, the lumbar curve, and the sacral curve. The cervical and lumbar curves are designed to curve in, while the other two curve out. When any of the curves flatten, the spine experiences distress, which can be managed with a consistent yoga practice.

8. *Describe the difference between negative pain, positive pain, and post-exercise pain.* Negative pain is sharp, jabs, bites, or burns and is typically located in or beside a joint. Positive pain can be a strong sensation, or a dull aching pain located in the muscle or tendons. Positive pain diminishes as we hold the pose, and when we stop stretching, the pain is gone and we feel better. Post exercise pain is a muscle soreness that mimics the pain of injury in the same location as the injury without any radiating pain and indicates a step toward strength and healing.

9. *Name four positive steps to follow when addressing pain.* When an intensity of pain or sensation is felt, *Stop and Breathe, Back off 10 percent, Suspend Judgment, Wait for the Release.*

10. *Name some facts you learned about fascia.* 1) Fascia is a web of connective tissue that comprises 20 percent of the human body. 2) It's on par in importance with the circulatory and nervous systems. 3) The pleating of fascia from injury or stress cannot be detected with any current medical technology and can limit mobility. 4) When we stretch, we also lengthen and organize fascia.

11. *How does yoga help relieve stress?* By turning our attention to long, deliberate breathing, the mind to the breath and the breath to the body, we reverse the stress cycle by releasing tension in the muscles as we hold poses and return the body/mind to the parasympathetic system.

12. *Where is the psoas muscle and what is its function?* This muscle is located deep inside the abdomen behind the organs, connecting the back to the front and the top to the bottom. Starting at T12, the vertebrae for the last rib, it attaches to all four lumbar vertebrae. The second half of the muscle forms the back inside wall of the pelvis, and inserts deep inside the groin on the inner thighbone. The psoas creates the lumbar and thoracic curves of the spine, flexes the leg toward the chest and the chest toward the leg, which makes it an important postural muscle and forms the inner two of the four muscular pillars of the spine.

13. *How does the psoas muscle contribute to back pain?* When overly contracted, the psoas pulls the pelvis to an anterior tilt, causing the low back to overly compress and the abdominal organs to protrude. In some bodies, only the long fibers of the psoas are shortened, in which case the lower ribs are drawn down and the thoracic curve becomes overly accentuated.

14. *Where is the pisiforms muscle and how/when in spasm does it trigger a pain response?* The pisiforms are a deep buttock muscle that externally rotates the leg. When overly contracted, it can press on the sciatic nerve, causing nerve pain or "false sciatica"—false because the vertebrae and discs are healthy and not pressing on the nerve. Gradual stretching in alignment to create release and muscular balance is the best approach.

15. *What is the difference between a de-stabilizing and stabilizing pose?* How does this inform our practice? De-stabilizing poses create mobility and are asymmetrical, meaning you perform the pose two times, once to the right and once to the left. Stabilizing poses are symmetrical and create balance—they have only one side. Downward facing dog pose is an example. I recommend you finish a practice with one or two stabilizing pose to integrate the mobility created by your yoga practice.

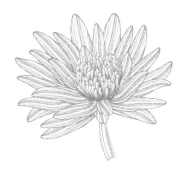

part 2

Building Range of Motion and Strength

Continuing to progress through the practice of yoga for back care, we move deeper into the muscles of the hips and shoulders, refining muscular balance to connect all parts of your spine, expand your range of motion, and build muscle tone. We offer seven sequences that address the hips, shoulders, legs, and spine—essential elements of a healthy back.

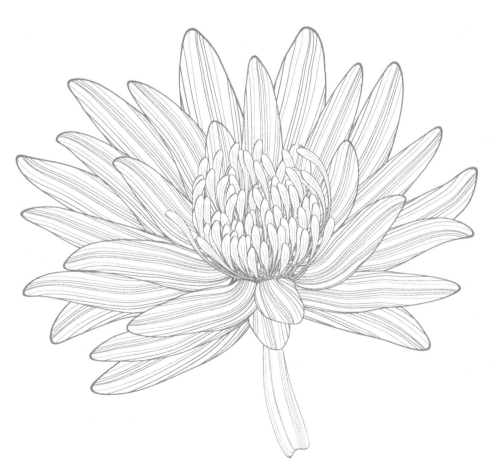

The Hip Sequence

In order to create mobility, ease, and healing in the spine, we need a balance of mobility and ease in the hip joints. Balanced mobility helps us in several ways: by creating a more even gate, an extended stride, and a more even weight distribution when we're standing. The implication is that we have the option to stand taller, allowing for more support and less stress on our spines, while also improving and maintaining the health of our hip joints.

As I described earlier in the book (see page 15) for simplicity's sake, there are three types of bodies—Ultra-contracted, Loosey-goosey, and Combo-pack. Most people find themselves in the category of the Combo-pack. The hip series I put together offers a yoga pose or stretch for each anatomical movement of the hip joint, which pretty much guarantees that no matter what body type you are, you'll benefit from these poses. With this series, you'll be able to identify which of your muscles are tight or short and which are loose or long. You'll also be able to determine if the same muscle on each leg is different, helping you to identify what your body needs to arrive at relative balance. *Remember that a muscle that has been in spasm when relaxed is always a weak muscle, even though its length remains short.* Therefore, observe

yourself both objectively as well as subjectively by noticing the range of motion in each leg compared with the sensations of instability or strain that would indicate weakness. Be patient, and give yourself the time to practice. Listen to your body and let your inner wisdom be your guide.

Even though our tighter muscles tend to hurt more when we stretch, they do require that we spend more time in the poses that stretch them, rather than in the poses that come easily. A simple way to monitor yourself is to use a timer when you practice. The general guideline is to hold each position for 15–30 seconds, which for most of us equals 3–5 breaths. Of course, our hamstrings typically require more time to lengthen, therefore, holding the leg stretches for 1–2 minutes on each side is not considered overdoing. Sometimes a muscle needs to stretch and sometimes it needs to build tone. Please be mindful not to overstretch a muscle that is already too long or gives you a feeling of weakness.

Note: In all supine poses, see that your forehead is parallel to the floor to avoid any strain in the neck, (i.e., avoid pinching any small or large tubes of the neck). When necessary, raise your head using a folded blanket so your neck and shoulders relax.

POSE 1. **STRAP STRETCH I / SUPTA PADANGUSTHASANA**

Practice all three positions with one leg before changing legs. The first version directly lengthens the hamstring muscles.

➤**1.** Place the belt on your right foot and take your right leg up as high as possible without bending your knee. ➤**2.** Press your left inner thigh down and lengthen the leg out through your heel. ➤**3.** When you exhale, extend the right heel toward the ceiling, as you inhale, draw down from the back of your right knee to the floor. ➤**4.** Maintain the balance of your clock face by moving the right hip away from your waist and toward the opposite inner thigh. ➤**5.** Hold 5–7 breaths (or 1 min on a side).

Hint: **Place a blanket under your head so that your forehead remains parallel to the floor to avoid pinching the tubes of the neck.**

Inner Action: Reach out through both legs as you extend your spine from the center of the clock face out through the crown of your head.

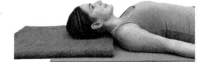

POSE 2. STRAP STRETCH II / PARSVA SUPTA PADANGUSTHASANA

This variation lengthens the inner leg or adductor muscles and further tones the lower abdominal muscles.

➤**1.** With the right leg up, hold the strap in your right hand. ➤**2.** Place the excess strap behind your neck and shoulder and hold it with your left hand also. ➤**3.** Place the block outside the thigh close to the hip for support. ➤**4.** Turn the leg out in the socket and draw it up toward your shoulder any amount. ➤**5.** Carry the leg out to the side while attempting to keep the opposite hip on the floor. ➤**6.** Receive the support of the block. Keep the outside of your foot parallel to the floor. ➤**7.** Extend the inner right leg toward the heel as you draw the center of your clock face toward the left. ➤**8.** Hold for 5–7 breaths.

Hint: Tone the gluteal muscles in this pose to help keep the opposite hip down on the floor. To do so, draw from the outer right foot and knee in toward the buttock as if to connect your thighbone to your tailbone. Extend from the inner groin out to the inner heel.

CAUTION: Lengthening the inner leg in this position is most challenging to your core strength—in particular the transverse abdominus and gluteal muscles. Therefore, I recommend you use the support of the block under the outer thigh to avoid misaligning the pelvis. This will help you keep 3:00 and 9:00 on the horizontal line when the leg is out to the side. Misaligning the pelvis also means misaligning the low back.

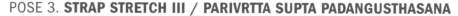

POSE 3. STRAP STRETCH III / PARIVRTTA SUPTA PADANGUSTHASANA

The third version lengthens the outer leg, hip, and low back, and stretches the abductor muscles.

➤**1.** Lie on the floor. Place the strap on the ball or back arch of your right foot, this time holding both ends of the strap in your left hand. ➤**2.** Extend the right leg out of the hip and carry it across your body, roll onto the outside of your left hip completely, and rest your foot on the floor or a block. Stack the hips one on top of the other so the clock face is perpendicular to the floor. ➤**3.** Straighten your left leg and spread the toes. ➤**4.** Extend your right arm alongside your head as you move the right hip away from your waist. Breathe. For a deeper twist, take the arm out to the side. ➤**5.** Extend your right leg any amount more by drawing back on the outer edge of the foot. ➤**6.** Hold this pose for 5–7 breaths and repeat on the other side.

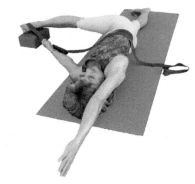

Hint 1: Be certain to move the top hip away from your waist to balance and decompress your lower back, keeping 3:00 and 9:00 stacked.

Hint 2: To stabilize your shoulder, draw the inner shoulder blade away from your ears, and turn the palm of your extended arm up as you slowly carry your arm out to the side any amount, as shown in the photo.

Inner Action: Lift the bottom of your belly in and up toward your chest as you press the center top thigh away from your chest to create more length in your spine.

CAUTION: If you have any pinching in your right (or left) groin, low back or hip, place a block under your foot, as shown in the photograph.

Note: However, when you first practice this pose, begin with the arm alongside your head to lengthen the spine and relieve compression. When your low back no longer gives you pain, you may increase the twist by taking your arm out to the side for the full expression of the pose.

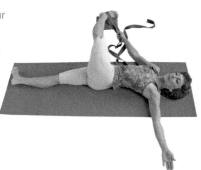

POSE 4. **TRACTION TWISTS A & B / SUPTA MATSYANGASANA**

Both versions of this pose extend the psoas muscles and tone the transverse abdominus, as well as traction the lower spine. See the Basic Low Back Sequence Pose 1 on page 23.

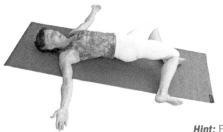

Version A

➤**1.** Place both feet on the floor, wider than your hips. ➤**2.** Drop your knees to the left so that your right knee is in line with your nose. ➤**3.** Extend from your outer right hip toward your knee, allowing your pelvis to lift up about halfway. ➤**4.** Curl the tip of your tailbone toward your pubis, and then draw the bottom of your belly in and up toward your chest. ➤**5.** Hold for 3–5 breaths on each side. Repeat each side twice.

Hint: Flex your feet to protect your knees.

Inner Action: Extend from your hip to your knee as you draw the center of your clock face in, up, then over to make the lower abdomen feel hollow, and move your right hip back toward the floor any amount.

CAUTION: If your right knee suffers any pain, please honor that and place a block under the knee for support—both above and below the joint. If any knee pain persists, stop doing the pose.

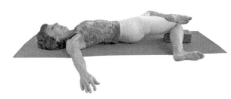

Version B

➤**1.** Repeat steps 1–4 in Version A. ➤**2.** Place a block under your right knee, supporting both above and below the joint. Now place the left foot on top of your right knee for a bigger stretch. Draw the bottom of your belly deeply in and up to keep your low back stable. ➤**3.** Hold for 3–5 breaths. Repeat each side twice.

Hint: If the block is limiting your stretch, then remove it, or use a folded blanket instead. If your knee and sacrum feel stable, feel free to work the stretch without any knee support.

CAUTION: Remove the weight of your left foot before lifting your knees back up.

POSE 5. **HIP STRETCH IN FLEXION / SUPTA AGNISTAMBASANA**

You may find the external rotation of the thigh in the hip socket, which uncovers the deep intrinsic muscles quite challenging, but this action is very important for the health of the hip joints. The pose presented here primarily stretches the piriformis muscles, along with the small gremilli muscles. Learn to let go mentally even when the physical response is not obvious.

Version A

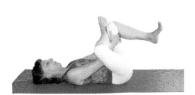

➤**1.** Lie on your back with knees bent, feet on the floor. ➤**2.** Cross your right ankle over the left knee. Keep your foot flexed and your ankle square to protect your knee. ➤**3.** Place both hands behind your left knee and draw the knees toward your chest any amount. ➤**4.** Use your right elbow to assist the right knee to point to the right. ➤**5.** Keep the clock face of the pelvis evenly balanced on the floor. Do your best to drop 6:00 toward the floor. ➤**6.** Breathe deeply into your hips and hold for 3–5 breaths. ➤**7.** Repeat each side twice.

Hint: It's important to keep the ankle of the right foot square to prevent any over stretching and instability in the knee joint.

Inner Action: Extend the back of your neck and release your shoulders toward your waist. Feel the length of your spine from the bottom of your belly through the crown of your head.

Note: Alternately, to keep 6:00 down, move near a wall and place your left foot on the wall so you have your hands free. Use your left hand to hold the left top thigh in place, and use your right hand to turn the right thigh out. Use both hands to keep your clock face balanced.

Pose 5 continued next page

Version B

Practicing this pose seated in a chair is helpful when your hips are very tight, or when you need a mid-day yoga break to relieve the stiffness of your hips.

➤**1.** Sit toward the front of the chair with your spine straight. ➤**2.** Place your right ankle on your left knee with your foot flexed. ➤**3.** Sharpen your sitting bones as you work to turn the outer knee toward the floor. ➤**4.** Breathe deeply into your hips and hold for 3–5 breaths, mentally letting go with each exhale. ➤**5.** Repeat each side twice.

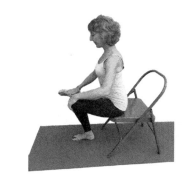

POSE 6. HIP STRETCH IN EXTENSION / UTTHITA AGNISTAMBASANA

Similar to the previous pose, this variation stretches the muscles of external rotation at their insertion in front on the hipbone, and also stretches the muscles that internally rotate the leg.

Version A

➤**1.** Begin sitting on the floor with your legs out straight. Place your right ankle directly under your left knee. ➤**2.** Place a block, blanket, or other prop under the right knee between the knee and the floor to protect the knee and hip from strain. ➤**3.** Lift your hips to tuck your tail toward your shin. ➤**4.** Place your left ankle on top of your right knee. Lean back as far as possible, or lie down on your back. ➤**5.** Draw the pelvic clock face in and up, and then attempt to drop your left knee down toward your right foot. ➤**6.** Hold for 7–10 breaths. Change sides.

Hint: Keep both feet flexed to protect the knees. As always, come out of a pose the same way you went in.

Inner Action: As you turn the top thighs out, lift your pelvic floor toward your breastbone to elongate the inside front of your spine.

CAUTION: Set yourself up in a good way so that your clock face stays parallel to the floor. This is the best way to protect your sacroiliac joints and low back from strain.

Version B

You may practice this pose seated in a chair so that gravity can help you release the tightness of your hips.

➤**1.** Sit toward the front of the chair with your spine straight. ➤**2.** Place your right ankle on your left knee with your foot flexed. ➤**3.** Lean back in the chair so you feel you're slumping. ➤**4.** Place your left hand on your belly, and with your right hand, grasp the inner right thigh at the knee. ➤**5.** As you exhale, simultaneously turn the right thigh out and down as you lift your lower belly in and up using your hands. ➤**6.** Hold for 3–5 breaths. Change sides.

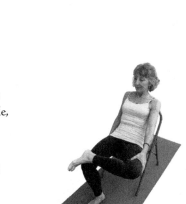

Hint: Feel free to move the left foot more under the chair seat to give gravity more of a chance to draw the right leg down.

POSE 7. **LUNGES A, B, C / VANARASANA**

Lunges are effective poses to help actively lengthen the quadriceps and psoas muscles. (See Pose 14 in the Alternate Low Back Sequence on page 42 for more details.)

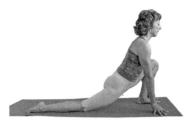

Version A–Low Lunge

➤**1.** Begin on your hands and knees. ➤**2.** Swing your left foot forward and place your ankle under your knee. ➤**3.** Slide the right knee back until you feel a good stretch on that front thigh. ➤**4.** Balance your clock face. ➤**6.** Hold for 3–5 breaths and change sides. Repeat again on both sides.

Hint: Turn the front knee out to squeeze that hip in toward your tailbone to stabilize your hips, further balance 3:00 and 9:00, and keep your low back extending evenly.

Inner Action: As you exhale, draw the center of your clock face in and up as you reach down and back with the rear knee.

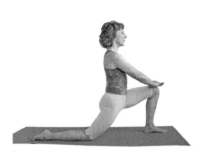

Version B–Low Lunge, Hands on Knee

➤**1.** Repeat steps 1–5 in Version A. ➤**2.** Ground down into your front heel and lift the bottom of your belly to raise your hands up onto your knee. ➤**3.** Balance your clock face side to side and front to back. ➤**4.** Hold for 3–5 breaths and change sides. Repeat again on both sides.

Inner Action: As you exhale, press the rear shin down and curl your tail again to draw the center of your clock face in and up. Relax your shoulders.

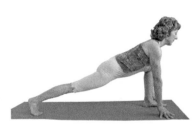

Version C–High Lunge

➤**1.** Repeat steps 1–5 in Version A, and then lift your right knee up to straighten the leg. ➤**2.** Make your right foot as vertical to the floor as possible. ➤**3.** Press the ball of the right foot down as you lift the ankle up to straighten the knee and lift the shin and thigh. ➤**4.** Lift the outer right hip so 3:00 and 9:00 remain parallel to the floor. ➤**5.** Extend the inner rear leg back as the inner front thigh reaches forward toward the knee. ➤**6.** Hold for 3–5 breaths and change sides. Repeat again on both sides.

Inner Action: Draw the center of the clock face in and up toward your chest equal to the extension back of the inner rear leg. Lift your collarbones to elongate your chest, with the neck in a neutral position.

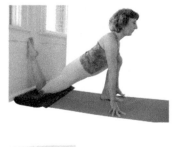

POSE 8. **WALL LUNGE VARIATION / VANARASANA**

These two lunges using the wall take you deeper into the stretch of the quadracep muscles necessary to sufficiently open the front of the thighs and create balanced movement for the hip joints. This version is recommended if you have problems in your knee joints or for any reason you are unable to perform the Half Reclined Hero's Pose that follows.

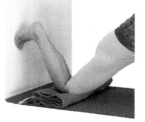

Version A

➤**1.** Place a folded blanket against the wall. ➤**2.** From a kneeling position, slide your left foot up the wall and place your knee on the blanket. ➤**3.** Swing your opposite foot forward into a lunge position. ➤**4.** Breath. Allow your hips to drop toward the floor as much as possible. ➤**5.** Hold for 5–7 breaths. Change legs.

Hint: For very tight quads, move your knee farther away from the wall and curl the toes of the back foot so the ball of the foot is touching the wall. Consider what it would mean to balance your clock face, especially 3:00 and 9:00.

Version B

➤**1.** Repeat steps 1–4 in Version A. ➤**2.** If possible, lift from the center of your clock face and place your hands onto your knee. ➤**3.** Draw your tail down to further lift your front hips. ➤**4.** Keep your hips away from the wall and the front knee bent as much as possible. ➤**5.** As you exhale press your foot into the wall and lift the bottom of the belly. ➤**6.** Hold for 5–7 breaths and change sides.

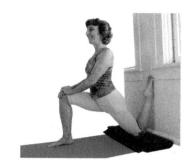

Hint: Adjust the pose by moving your hips forward and back to relieve the intensity of the stretch. Synchronize the movement with a long slow inhale and a long slow exhale.

CAUTION: Touching your hips to the wall places most of the intensity of stretch just above the knee. It's better for our purposes to keep the hips forward to lengthen from the mid-thigh up to the hip.

POSE 9. **HALF RECLINED HERO / ARDHA SUPTA VIRASANA**

This is the classic pose for releasing the quadracep muscles and resetting the head of the femur, or thighbone, deep into its socket. It's a wonderful choice if you can comfortably put your body into the pose and hold it for 2–4 minutes on a side. As this pose is a challenge for most people, please warm your muscles sufficiently beforehand; the deep lunges described above are excellent preparation. Choose this pose only if your knee joint is content, otherwise practice it first with the guidance of a knowledgeable yoga instructor. This pose can be done instead of or in addition to lunges.

Follow the same instructions for both versions presented here. The only real difference between the versions is the amount of height needed to make the pose accessible. Please note that when the hips are elevated, the height placed under the chest must also be elevated. The second photo shows the hips elevated on a block, therefore a bolster is needed under the chest. Additional height for the chest may be added using a folded blanket or an additional bolster.

Versions A and B

➤**1.** Begin by sitting on your heels. ➤**2.** If your knees are content, open your feet just enough to place your hips on the floor. Conversely, raise your hips up on a blanket, block, or both until your knees can accept the position. ➤**3.** Keep your toes pointing straight back. ➤**4.** Release one leg and place the foot on the floor. ➤**5.** Lean back on your hands, and then lift and slide your buttocks toward your folded knee. ➤**6.** Lie down on your back using the necessary support so that your folded knee stays on the floor. ➤**7.** Lengthen from the hip toward your knee as you draw your lower abdomen in and up.

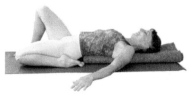

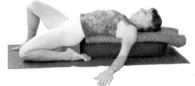

Hint: If your folded knee continues to "float" off the floor, place a folded blanket under that knee for support.

Inner Action: Point your toes straight back and spread them to draw your outer ankle bone in toward your hip to release tension and create balance in your knee joint.

CAUTION: Keep your clock face level to the floor by putting a blanket lift under the lower hip (the leg that is not folded under you). This will create balance in your pelvis and low back and prevent you from torqueing the ligaments of the sacrum.

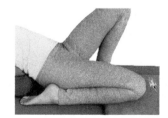

Note: Come out of the pose carefully, taking a few breaths to extend and flex your knee to relieve any strain in the knee joint.

Twisting Progressions for Back Care

Oftentimes, a back injury is caused by a twisting and/or lifting movement, resulting in torque and instability in the lumbar vertebrae that are involved. Consequently, chiropractors and physical therapists frequently recommend their clients avoid any twisting movements for an undetermined period of time. As reasonable as that request is, it doesn't address the necessity to return suppleness to all areas of the spine in order to create balanced movement and healing.

The twisting poses I recommend here have proven to be very safe for the whole spine, extending and opening areas that may be spot-welded together, while protecting the low back and more mobile areas. . You will find all these twists peppered throughout the sequences in this book. You may find one or two of these twists particularly helpful for your tight areas, so I urge you to practice them more often to give you the relief you seek.

There are three twisting poses listed below that are the most helpful as first-aid poses if and when you experience an aggravation of your low back problem. Your First-Aid Twists are poses 1, 8, and 11.

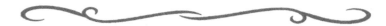

POSE 1. **TRACTION TWIST / SUPTA MATSYANGASANA**

This popular pose opens the psoas muscles and tractions the lumbar spine one side at a time.
See Pose 1 in the Basic Low Back Sequence on page 23 for more guidance.

➤**1.** Lie on your back and step your feet to the sides of your mat. ➤**2.** Drop both knees to the left. Extend out from the right hip to the right knee. ➤**3.** Curl your tail toward your pubic bone, as you draw the bottom of the belly in and up. ➤**4.** Hold for 3–5 breaths and change sides. Repeat 2–3 times.

Hint: Curl your tail so much that the bottom of your belly becomes hollow and your organs release and drop in toward your spine.

CAUTION: Flex your feet to protect your knee. Use a block under the knee as necessary for support.

POSE 2. **BASIC LYING TWIST / JATHARA PARIVARTANASANA**

Repetitions warm the body, tone the transverse and oblique abdominals, and release tension in the spine.
For more details, see Pose 6 in the Abdominal Progressions on page 36.

➤**1.** Extend your arms fully with the knees closer to your chest than your navel. ➤**2.** As you exhale and twist to the right, keep the knees 6–10 inches or more away from the floor. ➤**3.** Again exhale, and drop the lower belly in and turn your bottom ribs from the center of your clock face to the left. ➤**4.** Use your exhale to move in and out of the pose. ➤**5.** Hold for 1–2 breaths and change sides. Repeat 3–5 times.

Hint: If your spine is particularly stiff, you may place your knees on a block to stay in the pose longer. Add long, slow, deep breathes to release the diaphragm and open the chest. Continue to ask your belly to turn each time you exhale.

POSE 3. **YOGI CURL UPS WITH A TWIST**

This simple pose tones the upper psoas and oblique muscles. Refer to Pose 1, Version C, in the Abdominal Progressions on page 33 for more details.

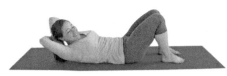

➤**1.** Lying with knees bent, hold your elbows in front of your chest, or cross your arms behind your head, as in the photo. ➤**2.** Exhale and curl up in the center, keeping the back bottom ribs on the floor. ➤**3.** Draw your left shoulder toward your right knee. ➤**4.** Hold for 3–5 breaths. Release. Change sides and repeat.

Hint: Keep the center of the clock face balanced on the floor as you bring each shoulder toward the opposite knee.

POSE 4. **SUPINE UPPER BACK TWIST / SUPTA MARICHYASANA III**

This pose releases and broadens the trapezius and rhomboid muscles, horizontally tractions the shoulder joints, and tones the psoas muscles. For more information, see Pose 5, Abdominal Progressions, page 38.

Version A

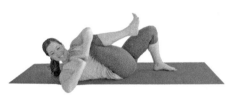

➤**1.** Bend both knees with your feet on the floor. ➤**2.** Lift your chest and hook one knee with the opposite elbow. ➤**3.** Press the knee out away from your chest and turn toward the knee. ➤**4.** Keep the clock face parallel to the floor and stable. ➤**5.** Hold for 3–5 breaths and repeat on the other side.

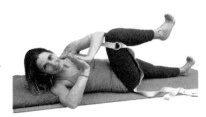

Hint: Place your palms together at right angles, and then lean on your bottom elbow to deepen the twist of the upper body.

Version B

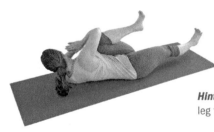

➤**1.** Begin as in Version A. ➤**2.** Straighten the opposite leg, hovering 6 inches off the floor or more. ➤**3.** Turn your chest further, keeping the clock face level to the floor. ➤**4.** Hold the knee steady as you twist towards it. ➤**5.** Hold for 3–5 breaths and repeat on the other side.

Hint: You can deepen the twist and increase the tone of the psoas muscles by broadening the back of the straight leg thigh and heel from the inseam out.

POSE 5. **SIDEWAYS CHAIR TWIST / BHARADVAJASANA**

Release tension in the small muscles along the spine with this simple twist. There's more information about the pose in the Basic Neck and Shoulder Sequence, Pose 11, page 32.

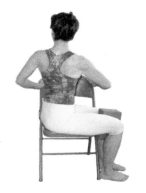

➤**1.** Sit sideways in the chair and place a block between your knees. ➤**2.** Lift your front spine from the bottom of your belly to your top chest and let your shoulders drop. ➤**3.** Exhale and rotate your spine from the bottom of the belly to the top. With each exhale, think to turn one vertebrae at a time from the base up. ➤**4.** Hold for 3–5 breaths and repeat on the other side.

Hint: Balance your rib cage. Keep the sides of your waist even so as not to misalign or stress your lumbar spine. Observe on which side the ribs are pushing out horizontally. Draw those ribs back in toward the midline as you lift the opposite side ribs that are collapsing. Also balance your ribs front to back keeping the "tube" of the spine neutral.

POSE 6. **OPEN CHAIR TWIST / MARICHYASANA I, SEATED VARIATION**

This variation opens the pectoralis major and minor muscles, releasing tension in the front and back of the neck.

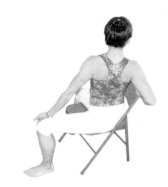

➤**1.** Place your mid-sacrum against the left side bar of a folding chair, with your legs apart at 90 degrees. ➤**2.** Lift your chest by moving your spine in and up. ➤**3.** Place your left hand inside the left knee, straighten the arm, and roll your shoulders back. ➤**4.** Bend your right arm and draw the elbow way back to place the hand against the outside of the chair back. ➤**5.** Turn your chest any amount toward the chair back to leverage your front chest open. ➤**6.** Reach your bent elbow back as you lift and press your chest forward. ➤**7.** Use the leverage of both arms to draw the shoulder blades down and pin them to your back ribs. ➤**8.** Hold for 3–5 breaths and repeat, moving to sit with your mid-sacrum against the right side bar of the chair and twist by reaching the left elbow back.

Hint: Extend your bent elbow diagonally away from your back so as to not compress the two shoulder blades together. Do press the shoulder blades onto your back ribs. Use your breath to help lift your chest.

POSE 7. **STANDING SCISSOR TWIST / PARSVA HASTA PADASANA**

This pose extends the front thigh, psoas muscle, and front spine as one unit to decompress the spine.

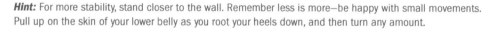
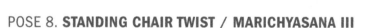

➤**1.** Place your hips close to a wall or counter for stability and leverage. ➤**2.** Step forward with the leg closest to the wall and back with the opposite leg until your legs form a triangle. ➤**3.** Actively press down into the rear heel as you extend from the back of your rear knee up toward your buttock. ➤**4.** Move your tail forward and lift the skin of your pubis in and up to elongate your clock face. ➤**5.** On an exhale, turn your navel toward the wall as far as possible, keeping the back heel rooting down. ➤**6.** Use the wall for leverage to help turn your chest. ➤**7.** Keep your nose centered over your breastbone as you turn. ➤**8.** Hold for 3–5 breaths and repeat on the other side.

Hint: For more stability, stand closer to the wall. Remember less is more—be happy with small movements. Pull up on the skin of your lower belly as you root your heels down, and then turn any amount.

POSE 8. **STANDING CHAIR TWIST / MARICHYASANA III**

The second first-aid pose is a standing twist that optimizes the length in the spine. This dual-action twist relieves tension along the spine by stretching the very small muscles that connect one vertebra to another, while building tone in the legs to help you gain length in your spine. Refer to the Alternate Low Back Sequence, Pose 16, on page 43, for more details.

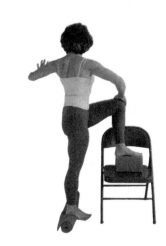

➤**1.** Begin by placing a chair against the wall with a block on the seat. ➤**2.** Stand beside and close to the chair with your heels elevated on a mat roll. ➤**3.** Place the foot that is closest to the wall on the block. ➤**4.** Stand in the back of your leg by aligning the center of your hip with your knee and ankle. ➤**5.** Lift your chest and spine from the center of your clock face, and then twist toward the wall. ➤**6.** With your opposite hand, hold the bent knee. Keep the knee stationary as you turn. ➤**7.** Imagine a line from your inner ankle to the crown of your head, and, on an exhale, turn your spine around that line, beginning with the center of your clock face. ➤**8.** Hold for 3–5 breaths. Repeat each side twice.

Hint: Anatomically, each vertebra only turns approximately 2 percent, so your aim is to distribute the turn along the whole spine. Also, if your low back is very tender, be sure to use a mat roll under the standing heel to further lift and decompress your spine.

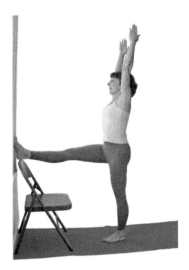

POSE 9. **STANDING HAND TO FOOT POSE / UTTHITA HASTA PADANGUSTHASANA**

Create length in the legs and spine, as well as strength in the legs and pelvic ring, with this pose. See Pose 17 of the Alternate Low Back Sequence on page 44 for more details.

➤**1.** Place your chair back against a wall for stability. ➤**2.** Stand facing your chair, one leg length away from the wall. ➤**3.** Place your left heel on the back of the chair or a block on the chair, toes touching the wall. ➤**4.** Align your standing leg from the inner ankle thru the center knee to the inner groin. ➤**5.** Move your inner groins back to the center of your pelvic floor, and then lift the bottom of the belly and draw the top buttocks down. ➤**6.** Squeeze in on the outside thigh of your standing leg to help stabilize the hips. ➤**7.** Then lift up through the inner leg and midline of your body to the crown of your head. ➤**8.** Extend from the back of both knees toward the buttocks to straighten your knees. ➤**9.** Raise your arms above your head and lift your palms up from the sides of your hips to extend your spine further. ➤**10.** Balance the clock face of your pelvis so the left and right hipbones are level. ➤**11.** Hold for 3–5 breaths. Repeat each side twice.

Hint: Be mindful of your standing leg and micro-bend the knee to avoid hyperextension of the knee. The alignment of the leg will give you more lift in your spine.

CAUTION: If you find balance to be a challenge, place the chair sideways against a wall before placing your foot on the chair.

POSE 10. **STANDING HAND TO FOOT AND TWIST / PARIVRTTA HASTA PADANGUSTHASANA**

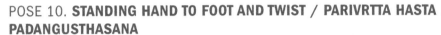

This pose opens the outer leg, improving mobility in your hips while toning the legs and your spine. It also aligns the spine by creating abdominal tone.

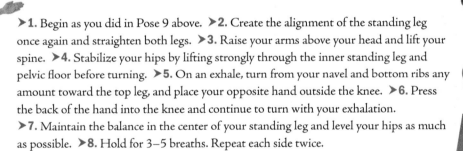

➤**1.** Begin as you did in Pose 9 above. ➤**2.** Create the alignment of the standing leg once again and straighten both legs. ➤**3.** Raise your arms above your head and lift your spine. ➤**4.** Stabilize your hips by lifting strongly through the inner standing leg and pelvic floor before turning. ➤**5.** On an exhale, turn from your navel and bottom ribs any amount toward the top leg, and place your opposite hand outside the knee. ➤**6.** Press the back of the hand into the knee and continue to turn with your exhalation. ➤**7.** Maintain the balance in the center of your standing leg and level your hips as much as possible. ➤**8.** Hold for 3–5 breaths. Repeat each side twice.

Hint: To avoid over extending the shoulder of the extended arm, press your palm into an imaginary glass wall, exhale to twist your chest toward the arm.

Inner Action: Lift an invisible line from the left inner knee up to the outer right hipbone as you exhale and turn.

POSE 11. **PRONE TWIST ON A BOLSTER / BHARADVAJASANA**

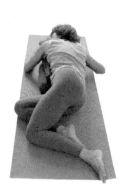

This third first-aid pose decompresses the lumbar spine one side at a time, creating space for a herniated disc to be drawn off the nerve and oftentimes inviting it back into place. You also can reduce low-back inflammation with this restorative twisting pose.

➤**1.** Sit on the floor with your legs folded to one side and your knees separated. ➤**2.** Place the bolster lengthwise 4–6 inches away from the side of your hip. ➤**3.** Lift your spine from the bottom of your belly. ➤**4.** -Exhale to twist your ribs, and then place your chest evenly on the bolster. ➤**5.** Begin by facing your nose in the same direction as your knees; turning the head to the opposite side is optional. ➤**6.** Hold each side for 1–3 minutes, breathing evenly.

Inner Action: Breathe into the spaces between your shoulder blades, as well as your lower back. Let go completely on your exhalations, softening your abdominal organs.

CAUTION: If you feel any pinching in the lower side of your waist, tuck the flesh of your side buttock under you and away from the bolster to relieve the "kink in the tube."

Anatomy & Key Muscles Affecting the Shoulders & Posture

Our shoulders and their anatomical balance are often a reflection of the position and balance of the pelvic and the respiratory diaphragms. Therefore when we align the pelvic floor by balancing the muscles of the hips and low back, we also create release and begin to re-align our shoulders. Please refer to the Anatomy & Key Muscles Affecting the Low Back on page 18 for a review of those muscles. The muscles highlighted here are the important ones to be aware of to release tension in the shoulders and chest to continue to create an upright posture.

Trapezius

The *trapezius* are large triangular muscles that form the upper back. Each side connects the seven cervical and all twelve thoracic vertebrae to the spine of the scapulae, shoulder blades. The trapezius muscle is divided into three sections—upper, middle, and lower.

➤ *Typically short:* the upper section has the most density and pulling power and is where we often hold tension by pulling our shoulders in and up.

➤ *Typically long:* the middle section is less dense and helps draw the shoulder blades toward each other. We often find those muscles long and weak from habitual rounded shoulders.

➤ *Typically long:* the lower section helps draw the inner shoulder blades down, often yielding to the stronger pull of the upper section, especially when the upper section is joined by the pull of the *rhomboids* and *levator scapulae.*

Rhomboid

The *rhomboids* are small muscles that lie under the mid-trapezius muscle, connecting the first five thoracic vertebrae with the inner edge of the shoulder blades. They form a triangle between the shoulder blades. They draw the shoulder blades toward the spine and also lift the inner edge of the shoulder blades up along with the levator scapulae.

➤ *Long muscles:* are typically seen as a winging of the shoulder blade. Combined with a weak mid-trapezius, they yield to the power of the pectoral muscles, thus contributing to rounded shoulders and posterior neck strain. Day-to-day activities primarily roll our shoulders forward as we reach out or down

with our arms and our eyes. These activities create length in the mid-trapezius and rhomboid muscles, causing the upper trapezius (top shoulder) to overly tighten. A focus on toning these muscles will help release tight chest muscles through reciprocal inhibition and help bring the chest back to the upright position.

➤ *Short muscles:* rarely occur except in extreme circumstances and injuries.

Levator Scapulae

The levator scapulae are small muscles that attach the cervical vertebrae 1–4 to the top inner edge of the shoulder blade.

➤ *Short muscles:* draw the shoulder blades and back of the head toward each other resulting in tightness and compression in the back neck.

➤ *Long muscles:* often reflect weakness and strain from to many hours with the head forward and eyes down.

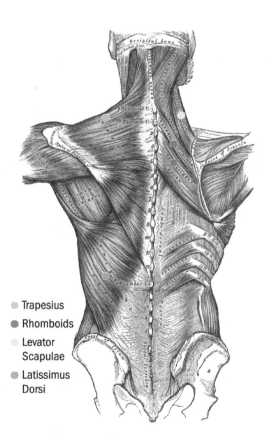

- Trapesius
- Rhomboids
- Levator Scapulae
- Latissimus Dorsi

Pectoralis Major and Minor

The *pectoralis major* are large muscles of the front chest that attach the sternum, collarbone, and costal cartilage to the front of the *humerus* (the upper arm bone) under the *deltoid* muscle.

The *pectoralis minor* originates at ribs 3 to 5 on the front chest, and inserts above to the *coracoid process* of the *scapulae* (shoulder blades).

➤ *Short muscles:* tend to contract the front chest and draw the shoulders forward. A collapsed chest creates contraction and strain on the posterior neck muscles, because we must lift our heads to look forward, which can result in forward head carriage.

➤ *Long muscles:* allow the shoulders to roll back and the chest to lift. An open chest is a prerequisite to be able to release the shoulders down, lengthen the back neck, and bring the head back into alignment.

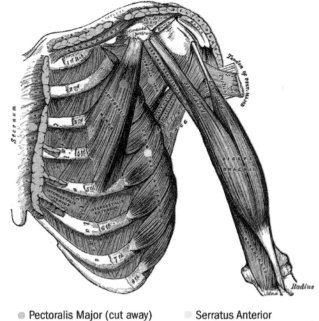

● Pectoralis Major (cut away)   ○ Serratus Anterior
● Pectoralis Minor   ● Subscapularis

Serratus Anterior

The *serratus anterior* is a broad, thin muscle that covers the lateral ribcage known as the "banana or finger muscle." The fingers originate from the upper eight ribs and insert along the entire medial, inside, boarder of the *scapulae* (shoulder blade). This muscle is responsible for rotating and stabilizing the shoulder blade when we raise our arms overhead.

➤ *Underdeveloped muscles:* leave the shoulder joint vulnerable to strain or possible injury to the rotator cuff when performing yoga poses that weight bear on the arms. This muscle requires development in yoga in order to extend the arms overhead with confidence.

➤ *Developed muscles:* draw the inner shoulder blades down and forward, upwardly rotating and stabilizing the blade so we can safely rotate the arm into full extension above the head without any pinching in the shoulder joint.

The Rotator Cuff

The shoulder joint is made up of four muscles called the *rotator cuff*. Known as the intrinsic or deep muscles, they surround and reinforce the *gleno-humeral joint capsule*, which is made of cartilage. These are small inner muscles that assist and limit the movement of the larger shoulder muscles. Also, when the large muscles become overly muscle bound or restricted, the shoulder joint itself becomes more vulnerable to deterioration, strain, and injury. In the case of a frozen shoulder, the rotator cuff muscles have become spot-welded in some combination, blocking shoulder movement.

1. **Subscapularis:** found on the anterior surface of the shoulder blade, between the blade and the ribs, attaches to the front of the upper arm.

   ➤ Actions: adducts or draws the arm toward the midline and internally rotates the upper arm along with pectorals major, ie; rolling the upper arm bone in toward the chest. This muscle also stabilizes the top of the arm bone when our arms are extended overhead.

2. **Supraspinatus:** originates above the spine of the shoulder blade, passes under the *acromio-clavicular joint* through a narrow space, inserts at the top of the humerus or upper arm bone. This is the most vulnerable muscle of the rotator cuff as it easily becomes pinched when we lift the arm sideways and overhead without externally rotating the arm in the socket first.

   ➤ Action: abducts or lifts the arm sideways to 90 degrees only. For the arm to go higher, the arm must first externally rotate, and then lift with the aid of other muscles—namely the *infraspinatus* and *teres major* muscles.

3. **Infraspinatus:** originates below the spine of the shoulder blade and inserts below the *supraspinatus*, just on the back side of the upper arm bone.

   ➤ Action: externally rotates the arm helping to broaden the pectoralis muscle of the chest.

4. **Teres Minor:** a short muscle that originates at the mid lateral boarder of the shoulder blade and inserts below the infraspinatus on the back side of the upper arm bone.

   ➤ Action: external rotation of the upper arm.

Note: The external rotators of the arm are small muscles that join with the rhomboids and mid-trapezius to counteract the pull of the pectoralis, subscapularis, and teres major muscles to help return us to our upright posture.

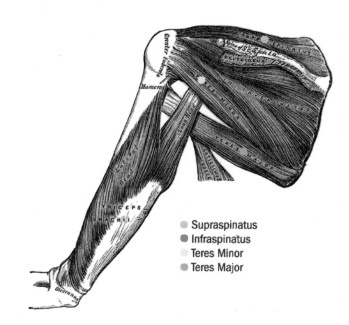

- ⬤ Supraspinatus
- ⬤ Infraspinatus
- ⬤ Teres Minor
- ⬤ Teres Major

Shoulder Release Sequence

As our body parts are inter-connected, it's not unusual for people who experience pain in their lower back to also experience some correlating tension and pain in the neck and shoulder region. Also, long hours sitting for computer work creates significant restriction in the neck, shoulder, and arms—sometimes even mimicking carpel tunnel syndrome. Once you have stabilized your low back and opened the deeper hip muscles, it's time to open and release the shoulder girdle as well to reduce wear and tear in the neck, arms, and hands.

Even though you may experience restriction, pain, and numbness in the forearm or hand, you may not have carpel tunnel syndrome. The many tendons and fascia in the shoulders and arms can constrict and press on the nerves causing irritation. Repetitive motion activities such as working with a computer mouse daily, consistently painting walls, playing a guitar, or participating in a one-side dominant sport, cause the muscles and fascia to contract restricting movement often pinching the nerves. Think of it as the small tubes of the arms being pinched and asking for release. So whether you suspect carpel tunnel syndrome, or simply find yourself with discomfort in your wrists and hands, you'll find this sequence helpful.

Honoring the intent of our yoga practice, the poses in this sequence are all intended to create length and space in and around the shoulder joint. Due to the anatomical fact that 80 percent of the nerve fibers in our bodies exist in the head and arms, when you experience pain or restriction in the wrist or shoulders, I recommend you practice this sequence. Progress slowly with these poses. At times it is difficult to separate negative nerve pain from positive muscle and connective tissue pain that might press on the nerves, therefore this Shoulder Release Sequence focuses on only non-weight bearing poses to create length, and space, to loosen the muscles and fascia of the arms and shoulders.

Sometimes a yoga student will experience tingling or a bit of numbness in the arms and hands due to the unavoidable squeezing of the nerves that occurs while stretching. If this happens to you as you practice these poses, back off 10 percent, breath deeply, and wait. Don't push. When you come out of the pose, the feeling should return to your hands within a few breaths. When you feel numbness in the pose, know that you're pressing on the fascia and returning it to liquid crystal from a solid state, ultimately decompressing the nerve pathways that run from the neck to the arms maintaining the function of your hands and arms.

Each of the poses in this sequence will help you release the small as well as the larger muscles of the shoulders and chest. As with the Hip Sequence, if you find two or three positions that address your tight places particularly well, feel free to repeat those more often. However, remember to practice the entire sequence also in order to achieve relative balance and freedom of movement in your shoulders and upper back.

POSE 1. **SIDEWAYS CHAIR TWIST / BHARADVAJASANA**

This first pose releases tension along the spine, making the spinal muscles more flexible while maintaining length and space. For complete instructions, see Pose 11 in the Basic Neck and Shoulder Sequence on page 32 and Pose 5 in the Progressive Twists on page 64)

➤**1.** With the block in position, and your sacrum vertical on top of your sitz bones, lift your chest from the bottom of your belly and roll your shoulders back. ➤**2.** Inhale fully, and on the exhale, turn from the bottom of your belly, pushing against the chair back with one hand and pulling with the other. ➤**3.** With each exhale, empty your belly and continue to turn, so that you experience the twist gradually from the lower vertebrae to the top. ➤**4.** In each segment of the twist, hold for 3–5 breaths. ➤**5.** Turn to face the other way in the chair, and repeat.

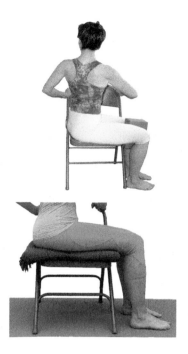

Note: In order to avoid collapsing your lower back, adjust the chair to match your height by placing a folded blanket under your hips until the center of your hip joint is slightly higher than the center of your knee joint. If you're short, place the blanket under your feet so you have a firm foundation.

Hint: Balance your rib cage. Keep the sides of your waist even so as not to misalign or stress your lumbar spine. Observe on which side the ribs are pushing out horizontally. Draw those ribs back in toward the midline as you lift the opposite side ribs that are collapsing.

Inner Action: Lift your spine with each inhale before twisting to decompress the tube of your spine.

POSE 2. **OPEN TWIST IN A CHAIR / MARICHYASANA I**

This pose is ideal for creating length in the muscles of the front chest and simultaneously helping to tone the muscles across the shoulder blades—namely, the pectoralis major and minor are lengthening while the mid-trapesius, and the rhomboids are toning. For more details, refer to Pose 6 in Progressive Twists, page 65.

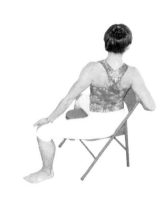

➤**1.** Place your mid-sacrum against the side bar of the chair, legs 90 degrees apart, and lift your chest by moving your spine in and up. ➤**2.** Place your left hand inside your left knee. ➤**3.** Bend your right arm and draw the elbow way back to place the hand against the outside of the chair back. ➤**4.** Draw the shoulder blades down and pin them to your back ribs. ➤**5.** Reach your bent elbow back as you lift and press your chest forward. ➤**6.** Hold for 3–5 breaths. Face the other direction and repeat.

Hint: Extend your bent elbow diagonally away from your back so as to not compress the two shoulder blades together. Use your breath to help lift your chest.

POSE 3. **EAGLE ARMS / GARUDASANA**

This is a good pose to release the upper trapezius muscles, and the levetor scapulae at the back of the neck. It both stretches and tones the rhomboid muscles. For detailed instructions, see Pose 9 in the Basic Neck and Shoulder Sequence on page 31.

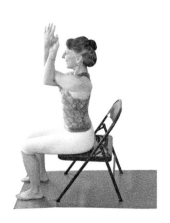

➤**1.** Sitting with your spine straight, entwine your arms as shown in the photo. ➤**2.** Keeping your elbows parallel to the floor, draw your shoulders down and apart. ➤**3.** Inhale to lift your breastbone, and then exhale and press your forearms into each other. ➤**4.** Hold for 3–5 breaths, and switch the position of your arms to stretch side two.

Hint: If you have very tight shoulders, you may not be able to wrap your hands in this manner. In this case, simply cross your arms at the elbows and keep the palms facing away from each other. As you exhale, press the forearms against each other to spread the shoulder blades.

POSE 4. **CLOSED TWIST IN THE CHAIR / ARDHA PASASANA**

Here's an excellent pose to tone the back of the arms and shoulders, release deep tension from the top chest and shoulders, and tone the spine.

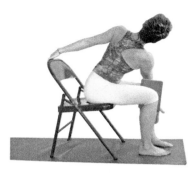

➤**1.** Place a block between your knees and sit toward the front edge of the chair. ➤**2.** Raise your right arm up to lengthen your spine. ➤**3.** As you exhale, twist and place your extended right arm outside your opposite knee. ➤**4.** Place your left hand on the back of the chair. ➤**5.** Inhale, to lift your chest and lengthen your front spine from the bottom of your belly out through the crown of your head, extending your central axis. ➤**6.** Exhale, press your arm into your knee to move your right armpit through and roll your left shoulder back. ➤**7.** Hold for 3–5 breaths. Change sides.

Hint: Turn your spine around the central axis by facing the middle of your breastbone directly to the left. Keep your nose in line with your breastbone so your eyes will gaze toward the wall on your left side when you have completed the twist.

CAUTION: Be sure to extend your front spine before turning to maintain length and space along the spine for ease of turning.

POSE 5. **HALF COW'S HEAD ARMS / ARDHA GOMUKHASANA**

The lower arm is isolated here so you can position the hand lower on your back to pin the shoulder blade to the back ribs. This action will deepen the opening of the small muscles that attach in the front of the shoulder. For the full pose, see Pose 10 in the Basic Neck and Shoulder Sequence, page 31.

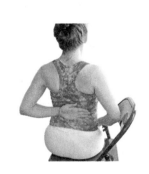

➤**1.** Sit or stand, with your spine straight. ➤**2.** Place your left arm behind you, with the outer wrist against your spine at the level of your waist or lower. ➤**3.** Roll your left shoulder forward, circle it up, back, and down. ➤**4.** Keep pointing your left elbow out to the side, rather than back. ➤**5.** Lift your breastbone. Breathe deeply. ➤**6.** Hold for 3–5 breaths. Change arms.

Hint: Press your thumb onto your back ribs and puff your armpit chest to flatten your shoulder blade onto your back ribs.

CAUTION: Rolling the shoulder back and pointing the elbow back are different movements. Avoid pointing your elbow back to remove strain on the front of the shoulder joint.

POSE 6. **UPWARD FACING STAFF IN A CHAIR / DWI PADA VIPARITA DANDASANA**

This pose helps to release tension in the small muscles of the shoulder joints and releases the diaphragm, which allows the chest to open. Releasing the diaphragm allows vital energy to flow more freely into the head, arms, and legs.

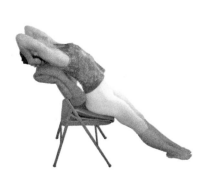

➤**1.** Place a double-folded blanket over the back of the chair for padding. ➤**2.** Sit in the chair, and slide your hips forward, and then lean back and drape the bottom of your shoulder blades over the back of the chair. ➤**3.** Interlace your fingers behind your head for support so your neck remains extended. ➤**4.** Draw your elbows in alongside your face to lift the outer armpit toward the ceiling. ➤**5.** Straighten your legs as much as possible. ➤**6.** Inhale deeply, and on an exhale, extend out through the points of your elbows to lengthen your side body and open your chest. ➤**7.** Hold for 3–5 breaths then repeat.

Hint: A tall person may need to place two blankets over the chair back to get the appropriate lift at the base of the shoulder blades. A short person may need a lift under their hips.

Inner Action: Wrap the outer arms around toward your face. As you extend out the elbows, draw the skin of your inner shoulder away from your ears to release tension in your neck.

CAUTION: Be certain to hold the back of your head so your eyes look toward the ceiling to avoid pinching the tube of your neck. Allow the bend to come from your chest lifting up onto the chair back.

POSE 7. **ONE ARM SIDEWAYS EXTENSION USING A WALL**

The channels of the arms are often constricted in various areas along the route. This pose opens the channels of the entire arm, stretching the nerves, muscles, and fascia to allow for greater ease.

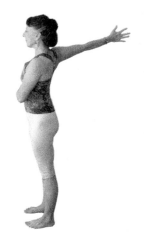

➤**1.** Stand sideways 6 inches away from the wall. ➤**2.** Reach your arm back behind your hip and place your palm on the wall. ➤**3.** Pin your shoulder blades to your back ribs and lift your chest. ➤**4.** Keep your arm straight as you walk your arm up the wall, pausing when you begin to feel the stretch.* ➤**5.** Reach back with your arm and fingers as you stretch your chest forward. ➤**6.** Continue to draw the inner shoulder blade down as you walk the arm up. ➤**7.** Hold for 3–5 breaths, and then change arms.

Note: *In order to reach the full turning of the shoulder blade and the lift of the armpit, work progressively over time to move the arm up the wall so it winds up slightly above horizontal.

Hint: Look to place your whole palm and all the fingers firmly on the wall. On an exhale, press the palm into the wall and extend out your fingers, to increase the depth of stretch and integrate the whole arm.

CAUTION: You may experience some numbness in the fingers or palm. This is par for the course as the tendons and fascia can easily press on the nerves. Remember, less is more, stop, back off 10 percent, wait, and breathe. Allow time for change.

POSE 8. **UPWARD HANDS FACING THE WALL / URDHVA HASTASANA**

Fully extend the arms in this pose as a non-weight-bearing version using the same arm actions as downward facing dog pose, see Pose 6B in the Basic Neck and Shoulders Sequence, page 30. Open the armpit chest, diaphragm, and ribs as you tone the serratus anterior muscles that are responsible for stabilizing the shoulder girdle.

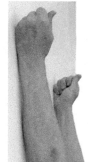

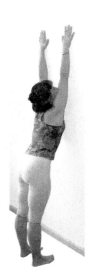

➤**1.** Facing the wall, stand 6–8 inches away. ➤**2.** Walk your hands up the wall as far as possible with your arms completely straight and parallel. ➤**3.** Rise up on your toes to reach higher. ➤**4.** Imagine your hands and arms growing long as you lower your heels to the floor. ➤**5.** Wrap your outer armpits toward the wall. ➤**6.** Bring your breastbone toward the wall as you draw your top thighs back. ➤**7.** Rest your forehead or chin on the wall. ➤**8.** Hold for 3–5 breaths. Repeat 3 times.

Hint: Sometimes the outer arm is difficult to wrap sufficiently as the serratus anterior muscle is often under-developed. In that case, feel free to separate your hands wider, as well as make a fist with your hands and press their outside edge into the wall to get leverage to draw the outer armpits toward the wall.

CAUTION: This pose offers an interesting dichotomy, as the tendency is to hang in the lower belly as the chest moves forward and up. Remember to protect your low back by lifting the center of your clock face without rounding your low back.

POSE 9. **BOTH ARMS EXTENDED BACK / PASCHIMA BADDHA HASTASANA**

The front of your arms are extended in this pose, along with the pectoralis major and minor muscles of the front chest. The back of the arms or triceps, the mid-trapezius, and the rhomboid muscles will be toned. The pose is similar to the Door Chest Hang, Pose 12, in the Basic Neck and Shoulder Sequence on page 32.

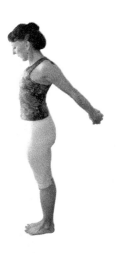

➤**1.** Interlace your fingers behind your back and Stand Tall. ➤**2.** Root your heels into the floor and lift from your front ankles up to your breastbone. ➤**3.** Roll your shoulders back and down to lift your armpit chest. ➤**4.** Extend the arms back as you reach your chest forward. ➤**5.** Raise the arms any amount. ➤**6.** Hold for 3–5 breaths. Repeat 3 times.

Hint: Release your head down to soften your neck and get more lift in your chest and arms. Breathe.

CAUTION: Lift the bottom of your belly in and up to stabilize your lower back.

POSE 10. **BOUND FINGER EXTENSION / BHADANGULLIASANA**

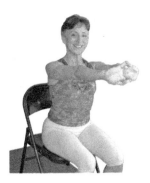

Stretch your wrist, fingers, and forearm with this pose to connect and lengthen all the fibers of the arms.

➤**1.** Either sitting or standing, interlace your fingers in front of you and flip your palms out.
➤**2.** Drop your shoulders down and raise your breastbone. ➤**3.** On an exhale, reach your palms forward, keeping your fingers and palms flat. ➤**4.** Draw your elbows in toward each other.
➤**5.** Hold for 3–5 breaths. ➤**6.** Change the interlace of your fingers and repeat.

Hint: Draw your thumbs down toward the floor and reach the webbings of your hands into each other.

CAUTION: If you are indeed experiencing inflammation in your wrist, proceed slowly. Remember to add lots of long, deep breaths as you progress into the extension. If you find this wrist stretch particularly challenging, please include it in your practice often to prevent any further loss of function in your wrists and fingers.

POSE 11. **REVERSE WRIST BEND SEATED**

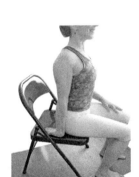

To balance and open both sides of the wrist and forearm, be certain to include this Reverse Wrist Bend every time you practice the Horizontal Bound Finger Extension above.

➤**1.** Sit tall in the chair and lift your breastbone. ➤**2.** Place the back of your palm on the seat as evenly as possible, spreading your fingers. ➤**3.** Turn the upper arm and shoulder all the way back to spin the elbow forward to the point of resistance in the arm or wrist. ➤**4.** Keep the knuckles down and add deep breathing to open. ➤**5.** Hold for 3–5 breaths. Change hands and repeat.

Hint: If your arms are proportionately long or short in relationship to your spine, try doing this pose sitting on the floor with your legs out straight, so you have more room to adjust your position.

Inner Action: "Spinning" the flesh around the bone presses and releases the fascia and small tendons of the forearm.

CAUTION: If your forearms are very contracted, it may be challenging to get your knuckles to touch the chair or to straighten your elbow, or both. As always, go forward as far as you can, and then stop, breathe and wait for the muscles to release. Muscles change and can be cultivated over time.

POSE 12. **FORWARD FOLD WITH HEAD SUPPORT / ARDHA UTTANASANA**

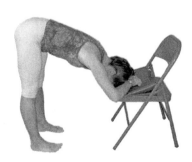

The final pose in this sequence is a forward fold to release your spine, neck, and head, and counterbalance the work of the shoulders and upper back.

➤**1.** Stand with your feet hip-width apart. ➤**2.** Fold forward at your hips and rest your head on your hands in the seat, or the back of the chair, depending on the length and ease of your hamstring muscles. ➤**3.** Micro-bend your knees to avoid hyper-extending. ➤**4.** Breathe deeply and relax you arms and shoulders. ➤**5.** Hold for 7 breaths.

Hint: You may place a blanket or block on the chair seat to allow your spine to round easily while stretching your hamstrings and releasing your spine, neck, and shoulders.

Inner Action: Move the skin of your forehead toward your chin to release all the tension throughout the spine and rest your brain.

CAUTION: If you feel discomfort in your lower back, step your feet wide apart to create ease and / or turn the chair around and place your forearms on the chair back.

Progressive Spinal Extensions

In many therapeutic approaches to back pain, extending the front spine is considered an important and even primary treatment. However, many students of yoga avoid spinal extension poses because they don't recognize their value, or know how to approach them safely, without causing negative pain. Anatomically we were designed to walk on all fours, which allows the spine to hang in a neutral position in relation to gravity. When we stand for long hours or sit in chairs, we tend to slump, and the spine compresses on itself. By using extension exercises properly, we can maintain an upright posture, openness in the chest, and strength in the spine.

The Progressive Spinal Extensions I recommend here begin at the lowest common denominator by first creating length and space in the spine, specifically using traction to reduce compression on the facet joints. From there, you can build gradually by opening the front thigh and psoas muscles with the various lunging poses, tone the upper back and open the chest,

and then tone the back muscles by curling the spine against the pull of gravity with locust pose, thus creating optimal weight bearing for the spinal muscles. Muscles love to contract because that's what they do best, so spinal extensions tone the back muscles to make them stronger and more able to hold us upright. Also the weight-bearing poses in this section have been used in research studies to demonstrate yoga's effect on reducing osteoporosis.

Once you've become familiar with the poses, this sequence will require approximately 50 minutes to complete. After you're able to practice these poses without any discomfort or negative pain, you can move on to other classic yogic spinal extensions, such as Camel Pose / Ustrasana, or Bow Pose / Dhanurasana, which are commonly practiced in general yoga classes.

In the list that follows, I indicate which muscles each of the poses will affect, and offer additional hints and inner actions for practicing them.

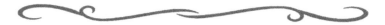

POSE 1. TRACTION STRAP STRETCH I, II, III / SUPTA PADANGUSTHASANA

This variation of the foundational pose series that lengthens the low back and hamstrings in part I, the inner leg or adductors in part II, and the outer leg and side body in part III, adds a second belt to create traction. Traction helps create space in the hip joint as well as decompress the lower spine, which is excellent for those experiencing acute back or sacral pain situations. Traction Strap Stretch can be used alone, or in combination with the Progressive Spinal Extensions presented here. You'll need two straps for these poses. Please refer to the Alternate Low Back Sequence, Poses 6, 7, and 8, on page 39 for more instruction about the three strap stretches.

After setting up the traction belt, practice all three legs positions on that one side, and then switch sides to repeat all three.

How to place the lower belt

➤**1.** Begin by making a large loop in your yoga belt. ➤**2.** Place it around the ball of your right foot and the top of your left thigh, deep in the hip crease. ➤**3.** Place the buckle on the outside of the leg so that it tightens toward your right foot. ➤**4.** Gradually tighten the belt so that you feel the pull of the thigh away from your belly.

Hint: If the belt cuts into your thigh, place a facecloth between the belt and the top thigh for padding.

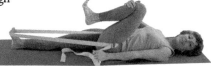

Pose 1 continued next page

Strap Stretch I–Leg up

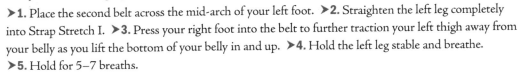

➤**1.** Place the second belt across the mid-arch of your left foot. ➤**2.** Straighten the left leg completely into Strap Stretch I. ➤**3.** Press your right foot into the belt to further traction your left thigh away from your belly as you lift the bottom of your belly in and up. ➤**4.** Hold the left leg stable and breathe. ➤**5.** Hold for 5–7 breaths.

Hint: Once the traction belt is adjusted for your current ability, keep the same length for the second side to enhance your awareness of symmetry.

Inner Action: Keep your jaw and throat soft, and perceive and receive the lengthening of your spine from your pelvic floor to the crown of your head.

CAUTION: Tighten the belt gradually and test your ability to straighten the left leg and still keep your clock face and spine neutral. Lengthen the belt in the left hand as much as necessary.

Strap Stretch II–Leg out to the side

➤**1.** Make a small loop in the second belt and place it across the arch of your foot. ➤**2.** Take the long end of the belt and pass it behind your neck, holding the tail with a bent right elbow. ➤**3.** Reach your left hand as far up the belt as possible so that your arm is completely straight. ➤**4.** Holding the belt with both hands, draw the left foot toward your shoulder any amount and then out to the side. ➤**5.** Remember to keep your clock face flat on the floor; use a block under your thigh for support as necessary to do so. ➤**6.** Extend out both arms and both legs completely. ➤**7.** Hold for 5–7 breaths, breathing evenly.

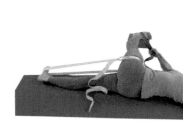

Hint: Allow the belt to remind you to move the left hip toward your right foot. Also draw your right hipbone up toward your right shoulder to help re-establish your clock face.

Hint 2: Lift the bottom of your belly in and up toward your chest as you press out with your right foot to further elongate your spine.

Strap Stretch III–Leg across the body

➤**1.** Switch the hold of the second belt to your right hand. ➤**2.** On an exhale, carry the leg across your body and place your left foot on a block. ➤**3.** Remember to stack your hips so the clock face is vertical. ➤**4.** Press your right foot into the belt to further traction your left thigh away from your belly as you lift the bottom of your belly in and up. ➤**5.** Hold the left leg stable and breathe. ➤**6.** Then roll your chest and shoulder open and extend your left arm any amount to the side. ➤**7.** Hold for 5–7 breaths.

Hint: If you take your arm out to the side, remember to draw the inner shoulder blade down and pin it to your back ribs so as to not strain your shoulder joint. Otherwise, leave your arm extended alongside your head.

Inner Action: Extend evenly out through all your limbs, including up your front spine and out the crown of your head. Use your breath to find your inner space, let go of resistance as much as possible, and then expand the inner space through your limbs.

POSE 2. **PELVIC LIFTS / SETU BANDHA SARVANGASANA_**

Previously you were introduced to two versions of active Pelvic Lifts in the Alternate Low Back Sequence, Poses 10 and 11, page 40. Here I offer you a third version that is more passive and supported to allow for ease and patience when you're seeking length in the hip flexors and lower spine. Guided by the results that will best serve the needs of your body at the time, choose any one of the three versions below.

➤**1.** Sitting on the floor with knees bent, align your toes with the edge of your mat or an imaginary line. ➤**2.** Slide your hips toward your feet so your knees are right over your ankles. ➤**3.** Lie on your back with your arms by your sides. ➤**4.** Choose Version A, B, or C. ➤**5.** Curl your tail and slide your knees forward to lift your hips. ➤**6.** Press your heels down to lift your hips higher. ➤**7.** Turn the upper arms under, shoulders blades moving toward the spine. ➤**8.** Press your arms down to raise your breastbone toward your chin in order to elongate your spine. ➤**9.** Hold 3–5 breaths.

Version A

Hold a block between the knees to tone the inner thighs and release the outer hips and low back. This version helps overcome the power of tight quadricep muscles by keeping the knees and thighs running parallel.

Hint: Watch for the sensation of the muscles. If you feel your low back tightening and your buttocks go soft, you have lost the length of your spine. Remember to take your tail bone deep in and lift your hips until you feel the resistance of your top thighs; stop there, even if you are only half way up. Hold for 3 breaths, and then repeat to warm the thighs and buttocks without shortening your low back.

Version B

Place a belt loop approximately 4–6 inches above your knees. As you lift, press out into the belt to activate and tone the gluteal muscles and move your sacrum deep in and further extend your spine. This pose is an excellent choice for persons who are overly flexible with weak hamstrings, sacroiliac instability, or bone density concerns.

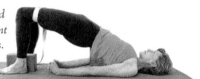

Hint: If the belt is around your mid-thigh or higher, your knees will tend to drift apart, causing the outer hip and buttock muscles to compress, which will narrow and tighten the low back. Instead, place the belt closer to your knees so your thighs continue to run parallel.

CAUTION: If you have any pinching in your knee joints, raise your feet onto blocks at the wall and/or loosen the belt to take your feet wider apart.

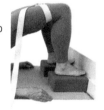

Version C

Having a block under the sacrum allows you to stay in this pose a long time, which contributes to the opening of the hip flexors, namely the ilio-psoas, iliacus, and quadracep muscles. After prolonged sitting these muscles become contracted, pulling the lower spine forward when we stand. Because it takes 30 seconds for the muscle spindles to release and 40 seconds for the fascia and tendons to begin to release, it's beneficial to hold this pose for several minutes, if you can.

➤**1.** Follow steps 1–3 above. ➤**2.** Lift your hips enough to place the block under your mid-sacrum. This is the same location as the mid-point of your clock face. ➤**3.** Without lifting your hips off the block, curl your tail between the legs as you draw the skin from behind your pubic bone in and up toward your chest to open the psoas and front hip. ➤**4.** -Continue to raise your breastbone toward your chin and soften your front throat. ➤**5.** Hold the pose 1–5 minutes with smooth deep breathing.

Hint: Consider also using a belt around your thighs to keep your knees and thighs running parallel, as in Version B.

Inner Action: As you inhale, think of expanding your diaphragm to lift your bottom front ribs from behind your pubis toward your face. In this way, you'll create length along the front of your spine, a necessary element of all spinal extension poses.

CAUTION: If you experience any pinching in your low back, find your way to relief in one of these four ways:
a. Curl your tailbone 5-10 percent more. **b.** Lift your chest and side ribs higher. **c.** Lower the block down one level.
d. Go back to active lifts Version A or B.

Note: The block has three heights. Begin on the mid-height before going to the tallest height.

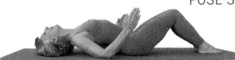

POSE 3. **HALF FISH POSE / ARDHA MATSYASANA**

Not only will this pose tone the upper back and neck muscles to relieve strain, it will also help open the top chest and expand the rib cage, which improves our posture. For complete instructions, see Pose 4 in the Basic Neck and Shoulder Sequence, page 29.

Hint: Be mindful to keep your spine long by lifting the space between your shoulders toward your chin.

➤**1.** Find the pose, as shown in the photo. ➤**2.** With your elbows bent, and 8–10 inches out from your ribs, turn the upper arms completely out so the shoulder blades lie flat between your chest and the floor. ➤**3.** Lift your chin until the back of the crown of your head touches the floor. Press the back of your head and elbows down to lift your shoulder blades up off the floor. ➤**4.** Extend the elbows diagonally down and out into the floor to draw the inner shoulder blades away from the neck and spread them apart. ➤**5.** Balance equally on your elbows and the back of your crown. ➤**6.** Hold for 3–5 breaths. Repeat 3 times.

Inner Action: With your inhale, simultaneously send the breath into your legs and your chest. Draw your organs in and up from behind your pubis toward your chest, as in the previous pose.

POSE 4. **LUNGES / VANARASANA**

The importance of opening the front hip in order to maintain spinal extension cannot be over emphasized. All three lunges from the Alternate Low Back Sequence, Pose 14, on page 42 are recommended here as a practice to warm up the front thigh after any amount of sitting, gardening, or hiking. Lunges help actively lengthen the quadriceps and psoas muscles, helping to increase the length of our spine by releasing the downward pull on the front of our hips. A balanced length of our hip flexors also allows our abdominal muscles to maintain tone and therefore support our lumbar spine. Because our bodies are dynamic, feel free to change the order of the poses; Version C could be practiced first.

Version A–Low Lunge

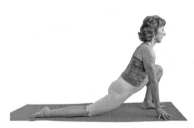

➤**1.** Move into the pose, as shown in the photo. ➤**2.** With your right knee down, slide the right knee back until you feel a good stretch on that front thigh. ➤**3.** Align the front knee with its own hip by turning the knee out and tucking the hip in. ➤**4.** Balance your clock face. ➤**5.** Hold for 3–5 breaths. Change sides, and then repeat.

Inner Action: As you exhale, draw the center of your clock face in and up as you reach down and back with the rear knee.

Version B–Low Lunge, Hands on knee

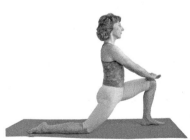

➤**1.** Begin in the Low Lunge, Version A. ➤**2.** Ground down through the left heel to lift your clock face in and up. ➤**3.** Raise your hands up onto your left knee. ➤**4.** Balance your clock face. ➤**5.** Hold for 3-5 breaths. Change sides, and then repeat.

Hint: As the tailbone squeezes forward, feel the pelvic floor tilt up slightly and the gluteal muscles on that side activate.

Inner Action: As you exhale, sink the front heel into the floor, curl your tail forward, and strongly draw the bottom of your belly in and up.

Version C–High Lunge

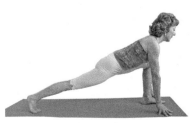

➤**1.** Begin as in Version A, and then lift your right knee up to straighten the leg. ➤**2.** Make your right foot as vertical to the floor as possible. ➤**3.** Press the ball of the right foot down as you lift the ankle up to straighten the knee and float the shin and thigh. ➤**4.** Lift the outer right hip so 3:00 and 9:00 remain parallel to the floor. ➤**5.** Extend the inner rear leg back as the inner front knee extends forward. ➤**6.** Hold for 3–5 breaths. Repeat each side twice.

Hint: Turn the front knee out to squeeze that hip in toward your tailbone to stabilize your hips, further balance 3:00 and 9:00, and keep your low back extending evenly.

Inner Action: Draw the center of the clock face in and up toward your chest equal to the extension back of the inner rear leg. Lift your collarbones to elongate your chest, with the neck in a neutral position.

POSE 5. **STANDING LUNGE / VIRABHADRASANA I**

The opening of the front hip and the extension of the lower spine from the previous poses will need to be integrated with the rest of the spine, so the spine can benefit from full extension. In order to do so, we need to extend and tone our legs. As I explained in the alignment principles in the introduction, the Subtle Actions (see page 14), when we extend to create length through our legs, we also create more length in our spine. To work your legs well, practice one or all three of these variations of the classical standing lunge. I recommend that you alternate the variation you choose to practice each time you do the sequence, even though you may have one version that is your favorite.

Version A

This version with the foot placed on a chair is recommended for very stiff bodies, as well as for situations where there maybe a bulging disc. Raising the knee helps keep the pelvis from collapsing forward, thus protecting the lower back.

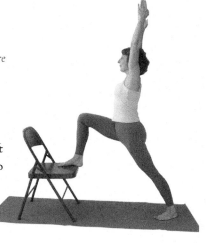

➤**1.** Place the chair against a wall, or place all four legs on a yoga mat to prevent it from slipping.
➤**2.** Stand Tall, aligning your inner knee, pelvic floor, and diaphragm with the crown of your head.
➤**3.** Bring your heels together and make a pie shape with your feet. ➤**4.** Now lift and place your left foot on the seat of the chair. ➤**5.** Root down into the outer rear heel of the standing leg and work to keep that top thigh pressing back. ➤**6.** Lift the bottom of your belly without bending the back knee. ➤**7.** Inhale, raising your arms overhead. ➤**8.** Exhale and lift the palms of your hands away from your hips to lengthen your spine. ➤**9.** With your next exhalation, draw the bottom of your belly in and up as you bend the front knee. ➤**10.** Continue extending as you hold the pose for 3 breaths.

Hint: If you need to partially lower your arms to keep your bottom front ribs down and back, simply extend out your fingertips as if to scoop your elbows up. Feel the extension of your outer armpit as you draw your inner shoulders down.

Inner Action: As you root down through the outer rear heel, lift up the inner leg into and through the pelvic floor along the inner spine, and connect to the lift of the chest.

CAUTION: If raising your arms overhead causes your back ribs to drop down and compress your low back, choose to keep your front ribs drawn down and balanced over your pelvis. In order to do so, you'll need to lower your arms to some degree. The degree varies person to person, depending on the flexibility of the shoulders.

Version B

This version, with the knee pressing a block into the wall, helps you drop the tail and draw the clock face in, thereby lengthening the psoas muscles and stabilizing the sacrum simultaneously.

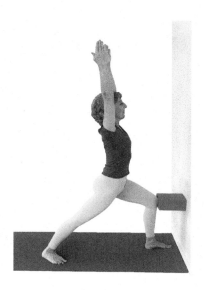

➤**1.** Place a block at the wall so you can hold it in place with your right kneecap, positioning your ankle below your knee. ➤**2.** Take a large step back with your left leg and place that foot so the heel is slightly turned in, like the pie shape in Version A. ➤**3.** Turn your hips to face forward, squaring the clock face toward the wall as best you can. ➤**4.** Press your knee into the block as you lift the right side of your pubis strongly up to balance 3:00 and 9:00. ➤**5.** Root down through the outer rear heel as you draw your lower belly back and up. ➤**6.** Inhale, raising your arms overhead. ➤**7.** Exhale, and lift the palms of your hands away from your hips to lengthen your spine. ➤**8.** Continue extending as you hold the pose for 3 breaths.

Hint: Maintain your base as you turn your hips. Keeping the outer rear heel down and the inner arch and anklebone lifted, slowly turn from your outer left hip toward the wall. Remember, the feet control and guide the hips. Shorten your stride as needed.

Inner Action: As you lift the bottom of your belly in and up, squeeze your outer left hip in toward your midline so you balance over your pelvic floor and activate the buttock muscles of the rear leg.

CAUTION: It's important to keep your hips in range, even if they're not perfectly square. This means that if you step too far back, your hip will move away from the wall and your lower back will become twisted, causing an imbalance in the muscles and resulting back pain. To correct, shorten your stride. Remember less is more.

Pose 5 continued next page

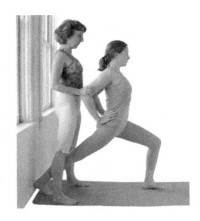

Version C

The version with the rear heel up on the wall is a good alternative for extending the back leg and spine completely when the calf muscles are short, there has been injury to the knee or ankle, or if the knee or ankle are tender in any way.

➤**1.** Place your left heel up the wall at a 45-degree angle. ➤**2.** Turn you hips to face forward, and step your right foot out as far as possible, keeping your hips square. ➤**3.** Use your hands on your hips to press down as you lift the bottom of your belly in and up to raise your chest. ➤**4.** As you exhale, bend your front knee any amount. ➤**5.** Continue to extend the inner rear heel into the wall as you lift from your pelvic floor to your chest. ➤**6.** Pause on the inhale, extend the leg, and lift your spine with each exhalation. ➤**7.** Hold for 3–5 breaths.

Hint: As you lift the bottom of the belly, the rear knee will want to bend. Maintain the extension of the rear knee and connection of that heel to the wall as you slowly bend the front knee any amount.

POSE 6. **DOOR CHEST HANG / URDHVA PURVOTTANASANA**

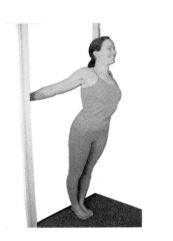

Open your front chest with this simple pose that you can access each time you pass through a doorway. It stretches the pectoralis major and minor, the bicep muscles and the forearm, and is an excellent choice after sitting for long hours, particularly when spending time at the computer. The full description is found in the Basic Neck and Shoulder Sequence, Pose 12, page 32.

➤**1.** Grab hold of the door jam behind you, as shown in the photo. Fold your fingers to a right angle and keep your wrist in a straight line to your elbow. ➤**2.** Lift and expand your chest forward as you draw your inner shoulder blades down. ➤**3.** Lean out with your chest and pin your shoulder blades to your back ribs. ➤**4.** Root your heels into the floor and lift from the bottom of your belly to raise your chest higher. ➤**5.** Breathe into your top chest. Hold for 3–5 breaths.

Hint: To increase the stretch, raise your hands higher on the door jam, or step your feet forward 3-4 inches. Feel the stretch anywhere through your top arm and upper chest below the collarbones.

Inner action: Isometricly press your palms out into the door jam to activate the muscles of the back arm and relieve pressure in the front of the shoulder.

CAUTION: Release any negative pressure on the inner elbow by micro-bending to bring more stretch to the chest.

POSE 7. **REVERSE PLANK / PURVOTTANASANA**

This pose extends the front of the arm and helps open the top chest. The muscles and nerve channels of the arm are extended, reducing pain in the thumbs. Because it's a weight-bearing pose, it will also build tone in the back of the arms. Here we find another example of reciprocal inhibition. When performed with a bent knee, the low back is protected and buttock muscles are also toned.

Hint 2: Keep your shoulder blades pinned and your top chest lifted, no matter how high your hips lift.

Version A

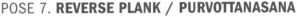

➤**1.** Sit on the front edge of a chair seat and place the heel of your hands behind your hips, fingers pointing out. ➤**2.** Roll your shoulders back and pin the bottom edge of your shoulder blades to your back ribs. ➤**3.** Walk your feet out, keeping the soles of your feet on the floor. ➤**4.** Inhale as you slide your hips forward and up, lifting your chest. ➤**5.** Keep your head level, eyes facing forward. ➤**6.** Exhale and return your hips to the chair. ➤**7.** Repeat 3 times. ➤**8.** On the 4ᵗʰ time, hold the pose for 3 breaths. ➤**9.** Press your heels down to firm and lift your buttocks higher. ➤**10.** Extend down into the heel of your hand to lift your side chest any amount. ➤**11.** Repeat the holding 3 times. ➤**12.** Rest.

Hint: If the muscles along the front of your arm are short, you'll find it difficult to lift your chest very high. If this pose proves to be challenging to you, all the more reason to practice it more often!

Version B

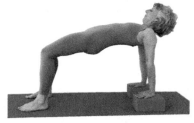

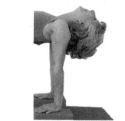

➤**1.** Sit on the floor and place the blocks at your sides just behind your buttocks. ➤**2.** Place the center of your palm in the center of the block for stability. ➤**3.** Roll your shoulders back and press your chest forward as in Version A. ➤**4.** Repeat steps 3–12 from Version A.

Hint: Before lifting your hips press your chest forward and extend your elbows back to relieve any pressure on the front of the joint capsule at the shoulder.

Hint 2: Taking the head back is the expression of the full pose and completes the extension of the spine.

CAUTION: Take your head back only if there is no discomfort or pinching of the small tubes of your neck.

POSE 8. **UPWARD FACING DOG / URDHVA MUKHA SVANASANA**

This dynamic pose extends the front spine from the pelvic floor to the top chest and tones the back of the body, making our spine stronger, and improving posture and organ function. It also helps tone the thighs and buttocks, improving bone density. Choose one of the two versions.

Version A

Choose additional support for the legs and low back with this version of upward facing dog pose. Placing your thighs on a bolster and your hands on blocks allows the belly to stretch and the spine to curl, toning the upper back muscles and minimizing compression in the low back.

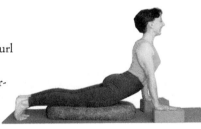

➤**1.** To begin, lie face down with your legs on the bolster and the front edge of the bolster across the bottom of your belly. ➤**2.** Place the blocks beside your waist, hands in the center of the block. ➤**3.** Curl your toes under and firm your thighs by straightening your knees. ➤**4.** Keeping the knees firm, press your tail down into the bolster. ➤**5.** Inhale and roll your shoulders back and draw your breastbone forward and up as you did in the door chest hang. ➤**6.** Continue to reach back through your heels and ground down through your tailbone as you straighten your arms as much as possible lifting your chest. ➤**7.** Hold briefly and repeat 3–5 times.

Hint: Curl the whole spine as best you can. Lengthen your front spine from the bottom of the belly to the bottom tip of the breastbone, and then curl the upper chest back.

CAUTION: For people with tighter shoulders and chest, you may need to work toward having your hands beside your waist. In this case, start with your hands beside your ribs and keep your elbows bent so you don't lift the chest as high up.

Version B

Placing your hands on the chair will help you passively maintain the length of the spine as you learn to develop the opening of your chest and the power in your arms and legs necessary to sustain an extended spine.

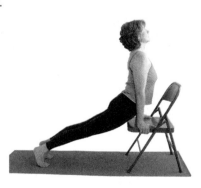

➤**1.** Face the back of the chair and place your hands just in front of your hips on the chair seat, fingers pointing out. ➤**2.** Bring your front hips to touch the seat of the chair. ➤**3.** Allow your knees to bend briefly to lift the bottom of your belly in and up toward your chest. ➤**4.** Roll your top shoulders back and press forward with the bottom tips of your shoulder blades. ➤**5.** Then reach your legs back and lift your inner thighs up any amount. ➤**6.** Extend back into your heels as you draw your tail forward and up toward your chest. ➤**7.** Breathe and hold the pose for 3–5 breaths. ➤**8.** Rest and repeat.

Hint: Roll your chest open from front to back by bending your elbows, pretend you're doing the door chest hang, and then straighten your arms and continue with the pose.

Inner Action: Squeeze the points of the elbow forward and lift up from the inner elbow to the front shoulder. Finish the loop, drawing the top of the back of each arm down toward the point of the elbow, to feel your chest curl open further.

CAUTION: If this pose stresses your low back in any way causing negative pain, try keeping your knees bent to make your clock face flatter, i.e., draw it in and up. If the pain persists, omit the pose from this sequence and consult with a knowledgeable yoga teacher or exercise therapist.

POSE 9. **DOWNWARD FACING DOG / ADHO MUKHA SVANASANA**

The practice of downward facing dog pose will return the spine to its full length and rest the spinal muscles after the previous two poses that have asked the spine to curl and tone. (For more about this pose, see Pose 6 in the Basic Neck and Shoulder Sequence, page 30.)

➤**1.** Keeping your knees bent, push up into the pose. ➤**2.** Press your palms into the floor to lift and extend your spine farther back and up toward your sitting bones. ➤**3.** Keep your heels lifted as you straighten your knees. ➤**4.** Reach the fingers forward as you press the top thighs back to continue extending the spine. ➤**5.** Hold for 7–10 breaths.

CAUTION: It's better to keep your knees bent and deepen the crease of your top thigh to extend your spine fully, than to straighten the knees and round the spine, which may create compression and discomfort in the lower back.

POSE 10. **LOCUST POSE / SALABHASANA**

Even though in classic Salabhasana both the chest and the legs lift, it's better to split the pose in half to avoid the fibers of the lower spine pulling into each other, which can shorten and compress those vertebrae. There are two ways to practice this pose. In Version A, you lift and curl the chest only, while extending the front spine so the spinal muscles can tone without compressing the vertebrae. In Version B, you moderately lift the legs to tone the buttocks and hamstrings. Practice both.

Version A–Chest only

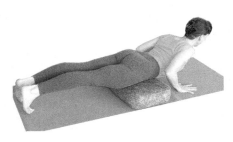

➤**1.** Place your hips on a bolster and your chest on the floor. ➤**2.** Place your hands beside your mid chest and curl your toes under. ➤**3.** Extend your legs completely, lifting your inner knees and thighs as you press your tail down. ➤**4.** Elongate from the pubis toward the chest as you draw your breastbone forward and extend your legs back. ➤**5.** Take your tail deep in as you curl your chest up. ➤**6.** Reach your elbows back toward your feet to press the bottom shoulder blades forward onto your back ribs. ➤**7.** Keep your toes on the floor and upper arm parallel to the floor. Hold for 3–4 breaths.

Hint: The more you extend back through your legs, the more you'll be able to expand your chest forward. Be aware of the less moveable parts of your spine and do your best to curl all parts of the spine equally.

CAUTION: Again, less is more. If you feel any negative pinching in your lower spine, back off by lowering your chest 10 percent. Anchor your tailbone more completely, and then continue to lengthen your spine, reaching your chest forward and your legs back.

Version B–Legs only

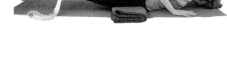

➤**1.** First, place a belt around your mid calf, feet approximately hip-width apart. ➤**2.** Lie down on your belly with your hips on a folded blanket and your chin or forehead on the floor. ➤**3.** Place your hands beside your chest and curl your toes under. ➤**4.** Lift the inner thighs up off the floor and then press your tail deep in. ➤**5.** Draw your shoulder blades and buttocks toward your feet, keeping the inner leg lifted. ➤**6.** With an exhale, lift your toes 2–4 inches off the floor, keeping the legs straight. ➤**7.** Press out on the belt as if to try to break it, in order to continue pulling the buttock muscles toward your feet and activate your hamstrings. ➤**8.** Hold for 3–5 breaths.

Hint: This pose activates all the muscles that hold the sacrum in place, toning the gluteal muscles and the hamstrings, and stabilizing your hips.

Inner Action: Extend out the heels as you pull up from the back of the knee toward the buttocks.

POSE 11. **WIDE LEG CHILD'S POSE / BALASANA**

Placing the knees wide allows the spine to remain neutral and not round so the disc spaces will remain even and full. Relax the low back and gluteal muscles in this way for a happy back. This pose is similar to the Kneeling Groin Stretch, Pose 11, in the Basic Low Back Sequence on page 27.

➤**1.** Take your knees very wide apart. ➤**2.** Begin with your hips forward toward your knees to bring your spine to neutral. ➤**3.** Slowly move your hips back and forth until your hips and low back relax. ➤**4.** Find a place to hold the pose without rounding your low back. ➤**5.** Place your forehead and elbows on the blanket. ➤**6.** Hold for 3–5 breaths. ➤**7.** To come out of the pose, slowly bring your knees together and then lift your chest.

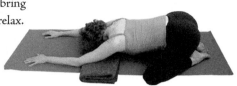

CAUTION: If your inner thighs are tight, keep your hips forward above your knees. It's more important to keep your lower back neutral than move your hips toward your feet.

POSE 12. **PELVIC LIFTS / SETU BANDHA SARVANGASANA**

This pose is similar to the more classic version shown in Pose 2 of this sequence. This variation provides an inversion that keeps the spine extended without compression and also minimizes weight bearing in the shoulders when compared to a full shoulderstand. The muscles of the spine and buttocks are toned and the hip joints become weightless. The glands and organs are naturally flushed, which improves their function, and the vascular system is toned.

➤**1.** Place the back of the chair against a wall to prevent it from slipping. ➤**2.** Lie down with your hips near the front legs of the chair so you can hold the legs with your hands. ➤**3.** Roll to your side and place a blanket under your shoulders and base of the neck to keep the neck from over flexing. ➤**4.** Roll onto your back once again and hold the front legs of the chair. ➤**5.** Place your feet on the seat of the chair or against the sides of the upper back. On an exhale, curl your tail and raise your hips up. ➤**6.** Roll your shoulders under you and toward your spine to relieve pressure in the head. ➤**7.** If possible hook your heels on the edge of the chair to prevent your feet from slipping. ➤**8.** Smooth and relax your breath. ➤**9.** Hold for 3–5 breaths and repeat 3–5 times.

Hint: As you drop your shoulders down, lengthen your spine up from your tail as if it were a star you were placing in the sky. Soften your face and neck.

CAUTION: If you have high blood pressure, even if it's controlled by medication, proceed with caution. Rather than hold this pose as recommended above, move into and out of it a few times, holding for no more than 2-3 breaths at a time, see how you respond. If you feel excess pressure in your face, head, or eyes, or shortness of breath, STOP. Consult with your healthcare professional before proceeding.

Note: Building cardio-vascular condition requires time and patience. Alternately, begin your practice of inversions with the Inverted Lake, Pose 5, found in the Six Restorative Poses section on page 49.

POSE 13. **CORPSE POSE / SAVASANA**

Version B—Calves on a Chair
(For more details, see the Basic Low Back Sequence, Pose 13 on page 00.)

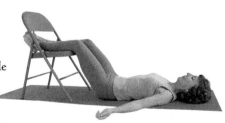

➤**1.** With your back flat on the floor, place your calves on the seat of a chair. ➤**2.** Place the middle of the back of your knee at the edge of the chair seat. ➤**3.** Let your calves rest heavy. ➤**4.** Stay in this position for 5 minutes.

Hint: Spread your spine on the floor and open the arms wide enough to soften your armpits. Let go completely.

Shoulder Toning Sequence

Practicing the sequences offered to this point, you've opened and balanced the muscles of your hips, low back, spine, and shoulders. Once you've created adequate length and space in your muscles and joints to re-discover ease of movement, it's then time to establish stability and strength by building muscle tone. The shoulders are no exception. By choosing to create stability and tone in the muscles of the shoulders, we are again choosing strength and resiliency to build an integrated spine. The shoulder toning sequence here follows all the principles of a good sequence by using several non-weight-bearing poses to warm and extend the muscles, affirming mobility, before asking the muscles to bear weight and thus become stronger.

You'll find this sequence invigorating and challenging. As always, breathe and lengthen your spine in all poses for the best results. The first 12 poses in the sequence have been chosen to give a deeper opening, space, and increased range of motion for the shoulder joints. You could stop your practice here when time is at a premium. Poses number 13–17 will build tone and strength, while the final three poses—18–20—will counter-balance the effort and return the spinal muscles to neutral. Initially, it will take you longer to practice the whole series; however, once you're familiar with the version of each pose that's working best for you, I anticipate the whole sequence will require 50–60 minutes to complete.

On pages 169–171 in the appendix, you'll find three different shoulder toning sequence variations at different levels of difficulty to choose from that require less time—30–40 minutes. As always, find the sequence that best serves your current abilities. Initially choose one of the sequences I recommend, so you can feel confident that you have a balanced practice.

Poses you've done in previous sequences appear here with a photo and minimal instruction. Look to the earlier sequences for more detailed descriptions.

Warm Ups, Poses 1–12 are all non-weight bearing:

POSE 1. **TRACTION TWIST**

(For more details, see Basic Low Back Sequence, Pose 1, page 23.)

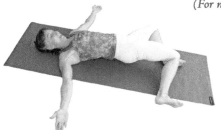

➤**1.** When you drop your knees to the left, be sure your right knee is in line with your nose: lift your head to check if this is so. ➤**2.** Extend from your outer right hip toward your knee, as you curl your tail in. ➤**3.** Hold for 3–5 breaths on each side, and repeat.

Remember: Keep the knee steady, and then curl the tip of your tail in toward your pubic bone, drawing the lower belly in and up until it feels hollow.

POSE 2. **PELVIC LIFTS / SETU BANDHA SARVANGASANA**

(For more details, see Alternate Low Back Sequence, Pose 10, Version A, page 40.)

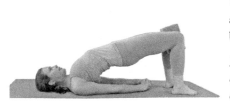

➤**1.** Move into the pose as shown in the photo. ➤**2.** Once the block is in place, curl your tail and slide your knees forward to lift your hips. ➤**3.** Turn the upper arms under your chest, shoulders blades moving toward the spine. ➤**4.** Repeat the lift 3 times, holding for 3–5 breaths.

Remember: Sink your heels to lift your hips and your tailbone. Also, press your arms down to raise your breastbone toward your chin in order to elongate your spine and extend/protect your lower back.

POSE 3. **HALF FISH POSE / ARDHA MATSYASANA**

(For more details, see Basic Neck and Shoulders Sequence, Pose 4, page 29.)

➤**1.** Move into the pose. ➤**2.** Be sure to press the back of your head and elbows down to engage the muscles of your upper back and neck to lift your chest up, forming an even arc from the top of the neck to the bottom of your shoulder blades. ➤**3.** Hold for 3–5 breaths. Repeat 3 times

Remember: Balance on your elbows and the back of your crown. Press the elbows diagonally into the floor to draw the inner shoulder blades down away from the neck and to also spread them apart.

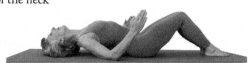

POSE 4. **SEATED CLOSED TWIST / MARICHYASANA III**

In Version A of this pose, the muscles of the spine, ribs, and shoulders are asked to become more flexible. The incremental turning of the spine around its axis increases mobility in the small muscles between the vertebrae. Also, the hamstring and deep, hip muscles of the bent knee will be stretched.

The additional affect of Version B is to tone the weaker muscles of the upper back, namely the mid-trapesius, rhomboids, and serratus anterior muscles, thus releasing the tight muscles of the front chest through reciprocal inhibition.

Version A

➤**1.** Sit on a bolster or two folded blankets in order to lift your spine straight. ➤**2.** Extend your legs out straight, feet together, as you have done in other poses. Bend your right knee and bring the heel toward the buttocks, stopping when the toes are even with the knee joint. ➤**3.** Slightly move your right hip back to make an angle. ➤**4.** Use your right hand behind you to press down and help you lift your spine. ➤**5.** Extend your left arm overhead, inhale, and raise the arm up out of the waist. ➤**6.** As you exhale, draw the bottom of your belly in and turn it as far as possible to the right. ➤**7.** Capture the right knee with your left elbow. ➤**8.** Progressively, with each exhalation, turn your spine—first the lower ribs, then the middle, then the upper ribs. ➤**9.** Work in the pose for 5–7 breaths. Change sides.

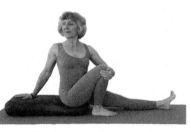

Inner Action: Squeeze the outer left hip toward your right groin to bring your left ribs toward your right thigh and stabilize the twist.

CAUTION: If one section of your spine is highly mobile, easily misaligning and causing pain, use caution in turning. Lift your spine more to create length and space first, and then slowly turn your spine. Again less is more.

Hint: Always begin turning from the bottom of your belly and work your way up your spine. The head should follow the spine, not lead; therefore, it should turn last.

Version B

➤**1.** Repeat steps 1–7 from Version A. ➤**2.** Cross your left arm over to place your elbow outside of your right knee. ➤**3.** Keep your right knee vertical and stable. ➤**4.** As you inhale, move your kidneys in and up, and roll your front shoulders back. ➤**5.** As you exhale, press your arm into your knee and your knee into your arm to turn. ➤**6.** Move your left armpit forward across your right thigh as you turn your right shoulder back, to further turn your mid and top ribs. ➤**7.** Turn your head any amount to gaze back. ➤**8.** Hold for 3–5 breaths. Change sides.

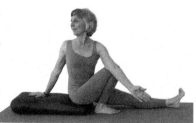

Hint: Always do your best to move your spine in and up and roll your shoulders back. See if you can turn from the more un-moveable parts of your spine in order to find balanced flexibility. Be Patient. Breathe.

Hint 2: If you have short hamstrings, are very tall, or for any reason have difficulty lifting your spine, put a block on top of the bolster or on the floor behind it. Lean back and place your right hand on the block and use it for leverage to create lift in your spine. When crossing your left arm to the outside of your right knee, make contact anywhere along your arm.

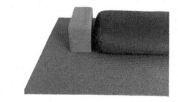

CAUTION: This seated twist is not recommended if you're having low back pain that is higher than a number 3 on the pain scale of 1–10 as it may create more instability in the low back.

POSE 5. **SEATED OPEN TWIST / MARICHYASANA I**

An open twist helps build tone in both the long and short fibers of the spine, the weak muscles of the upper back (as does Pose 4), and opens the front chest, from shoulder to shoulder.

Version A will activate the muscles of the back shoulder and armpit, namely the mid-trapezius, rhomboids, and serratus anterior muscles. Version B will give stability and traction to the shoulder joint as well as a point of reference by using the strap to more easily lift the spine in and up.

Version A

➤**1.** Begin as you did in the previous twist, sitting on a bolster or two folded blankets, with your legs straight. ➤**2.** Bend your left knee and place your foot in line with the center of your buttocks. ➤**3.** Keep your hips square, facing straight ahead. ➤**4.** Take your right arm back behind you and press down to support the lift of your spine. ➤**5.** Inhale and raise the left arm up as if you're lifting it out of your waist. ➤**6.** Exhale, empty your belly of breath, and then turn your spine from the bottom of your belly to the right. ➤**7.** Place your left arm inside your left knee. ➤**8.** Holding your left knee vertical and stationary, press the arm against the knee to move your left armpit to the right. ➤**9.** Roll your front shoulders back and keep pressing both sitting bones evenly down. ➤**10.** Gaze at your right foot. ➤**11.** Hold for 3–5 breaths. Change sides.

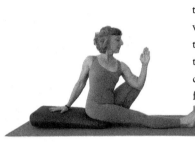

> **Hint:** Work to lift and elongate your front spine by moving your kidneys in and up toward your top chest, and then continue to turn.

Inner Action: Turn your right ribs back around toward the left and your left ribs forward and around toward the right.

Version B

➤**1.** Repeat steps 1–6 from Version A. ➤**2.** Hinge at your hips to reach forward toward your straight leg as if to touch your toes. ➤**3.** Place a belt around your foot and hold the belt with a straight left arm. ➤**4.** Connect some portion of your left arm and shoulder to your inner left knee. ➤**5.** Move your spine in and up any amount to lengthen it, and then roll your shoulders back. ➤**6.** As you exhale, squeeze your left knee and hip toward your right groin to turn your shoulders. ➤**7.** Pause and deep breathe, giving your body a chance to open up. ➤**8.** Gaze at the foot of your straight leg. ➤**9.** Hold for 3–5 breaths, and then change sides.

Hint: As the shoulders are connected to your foot with the aid of the belt, roll your right shoulder further back until you create a sense of traction through your left shoulder.

> **Inner Action:** As you turn your right shoulder back, press out into the belt with the ball of your foot and lift your bottom ribs any amount.

CAUTION: Remember that the spine needs to lengthen in both the front and the back, therefore be careful to not over reach for your foot and collapse your front spine. Check to see that there is no strain in your lower back.

POSE 6. **HALF BOUND EASY TWIST / ARDHA BADDHA SUKHASANA**

This pose gives us access to stretch the small deep muscles of the shoulder joint, particularly the infraspinatus and subscapularis muscles, along with the pectoralis minor and the anterior deltoid.

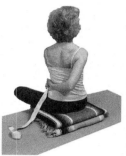
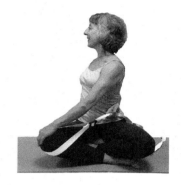

➤ **1.** Begin sitting on one or two blankets with your legs out straight. ➤ **2.** Fold your left leg in, followed by your right, so your right shin is in front. ➤ **3.** Place a belt loop around your right knee and hold the belt taught with your left hand. ➤ **4.** Lean forward slightly to wrap your right arm as far around your back toward your right knee as possible. ➤ **5.** Clasp the belt with your right hand and release the left hand. ➤ **6.** Sit up straight, and then turn to the right and hold onto your right knee with your left hand. ➤ **7.** Inhale and lift your spine. As you exhale, pull with your left hand to turn any amount. ➤ **8.** Hold for 3–5 breaths. ➤ **9.** Change the cross of your legs and twist in the other direction.

Hint: Sit high enough that you can easily lift your lower spine.

CAUTION: This is a deep stretch for the bound arm so remember to breathe deeply. If the bound arm goes numb, stop this pose for now and return to and practice the Shoulder Release Sequence on page 70, especially Poses 2, 5, 7, and 9.

POSE 7. **UPWARD BOUND FINGER EXTENSION / URDHVA BADDHANGULLYASANA**

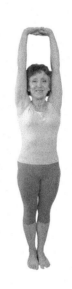

➤ **1.** Standing tall, interlace your fingers, turn your palms out, and extend your arms in front of you. ➤ **2.** Lift your breastbone as you draw your shoulder blades down away from your neck. ➤ **3.** Extend your arms forward to separate your shoulder blades, and then raise your arms up. ➤ **4.** Keeping your elbows straight, raise your arms as high as possible without disturbing your rib cage. ➤ **5.** Hold for 3 breaths. Lower your arms and repeat. ➤ **6.** Change the interlace of your fingers and repeat twice.

Hint: Lift your arms as high as possible without bending the elbows and work there to create openness. When the arms begin to loosen, you'll be able to raise them higher.

Inner Action: Continue to elongate and extend out the inner arm as you draw down from the outer elbow to the outer armpit.

CAUTION: As always, if you feel what you think may be negative pain, back out of the pose 10 percent, wait and breathe; something will begin to let go.

POSE 8. **EAGLE ARMS / GARUDASANA**

(For more details, refer to Basic Neck and Shoulder Sequence, Pose 9, page 31.)

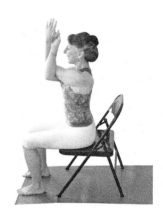

➤ **1.** Cross the left arm under the right at the elbow. Keep the right palm facing left. ➤ **2.** Wrap the right palm around to the little finger side of the left hand. ➤ **3.** With the upper arms parallel to the floor, drop your shoulder blades and lift your breastbone. ➤ **4.** Hold for 3–5 breaths on each side, and repeat.

Remember: If your shoulders are very tight, you may not be able to wrap your hands as shown. In this case, simply keep the palms facing away from each other and press the forearms into each other to drop and separate the shoulder blades.

Inner Action: Soften your throat as you move your shoulders down and apart.

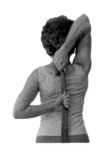

POSE 9. **COW'S HEAD ARMS / GOMUKHASANA**

(For more details, refer to Basic Neck and Shoulder Sequence, Pose 10, page 31.)

➤**1.** Place your left arm behind you, with the outer wrist against your spine at the level of your waist. ➤**2.** Roll your shoulder forward, up, back, and down, while pointing your elbow out to the side. ➤**3.** Lift your breastbone. ➤**4.** Take your right arm up alongside your head and drop your top hand down to grab the opposite fingers, or hold a strap between your hands.

Remember: Keep the top elbow wrapping in toward your head. Also press the wrist of the lower hand into your back and up to help you pin that shoulder blade to your back ribs.

Inner action: Elongate your breath and balance the sides of your ribcage.

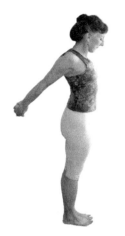

POSE 10. **BOTH ARMS EXTENDED BACK / PASCHIMA BADDHA HASTASANA**

(For more details, see Shoulder Release Sequence, Pose 9, page 73.)

➤**1.** Root your heels into the floor and lift from your front ankles up to your breastbone. ➤**2.** Roll your shoulders back and down to lift your armpit chest. ➤**3.** Extend the arms back as you reach your chest forward.

Remember: Extend both arms behind your back and lift them as high as possible toward the ceiling. Keep your fingers interlaced, palms facing in.

Inner Action: Inhale to lift your chest strongly up, and lower your head slightly to gaze down and soften your neck as your raise your arms.

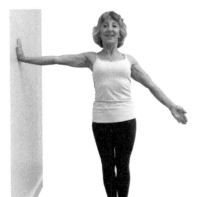

POSE 11. **SIDEWAYS WRIST STRETCH / URDHVA VASISTHASANA**

This pose does an amazing job of connecting to all the stuck fascia in the many tendons of our arms, opening the nerve pathways from the neck to the hands to help maintain the good functioning of our thumbs. Remember, the way to return fascia to the "gel" or fluid state is done through pressure, which this simple pose accomplishes.

➤**1.** Stand Tall, arms-distance from the wall beside you. ➤**2.** Place your hand on the wall so your wrist is level to your shoulders. ➤**3.** Press your whole palm into the wall as you roll your shoulder back and bring your armpit forward. ➤**4.** Revolve the skin of your arm from front to back at every inch along your arm. ➤**5.** Continue to press your whole palm into the wall as you draw your side ribs away. ➤**6.** Hold for 3–5 breaths, and then change sides.

Hint: Keep the bottom of your belly and chest lifted as you turn the skin of your arm.

CAUTION: If your wrist is very stiff or you feel any negative pain, adjust your position by raising your palm slightly higher than your shoulders, with your fingers pointing up, or lower than your shoulders, with your fingers pointing down.

Note: For even more benefit, repeat the stretch with your palm in 3 positions: fingers straight up, pointing back at 90 degrees, and pointing down toward the floor.

POSE 12. ARMS OVERHEAD WITH A POLE / URDHVA HASTASANA VARIATION

➤**1.** Stand Tall, and hold a broomstick pole in your hands, with your arms wide. ➤**2.** Raise your arms above your head. ➤**3.** Turn your arms in the sockets so the bottom of your armpits moves forward and the top of your arms turn back. ➤**4.** Root down through your heels, and lift the bottom of your belly up to lift your chest. ➤**5.** Keep turning the shoulders as you reach the arms back any amount to open your chest muscles. ➤**6.** Keep the elbows straight and the arms reaching toward your hands. ➤**7.** Breathe deeply into your top chest. ➤**8.** Hold for 5–7 breaths.

Hint: You will know when you have rotated your top arm back far enough because the sides of your neck will feel long and without tension. Tension in your neck is a reflection of the shoulders not turning enough or evenly. Try looking in a mirror to observe if both of your arms have rotated fully and evenly.

CAUTION: Be attentive to your wrist. If you feel any strain, hold the pole between your thumb and index finger only.

Poses 13–17 are all weight-bearing poses:

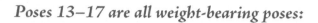

POSE 13. DOWNWARD FACING DOG / ADHO MUKHA SVANASANA

Choose to place your feet on the floor or on blocks at the wall, Version B or C. In Version B, the hands and feet are on the ground. In Version C the feet are up on blocks at the wall. (For more details, see Alternate Low Back Sequence, Poses 13 and 15, pages 41 and 43.)

➤**1.** From a kneeling position, place the palms ahead of your shoulders. ➤**2.** As usual, press your hands down to lift your hips into the air. ➤**3.** Move your pubic bone back between your legs to lift your hips further up. ➤**4.** Slowly straighten your knees. ➤**5.** Hold for 3–5 breaths.

Remember: Begin the pose with your knees bent to lift your hips, deepen the crease at the top of your thighs, and extend your spine. Maintaining the length of your spine, slowly straighten your knees.

Inner Action: Reach the whole palm down into the floor as you lengthen the inner arm and shoulder all the way up to your hips. Take the middle of your thighbone back.

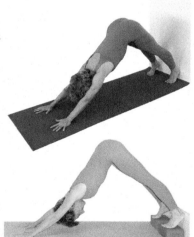

POSE 14. LOCUST POSE / SALABHASANA

Each of the variations shown will progressively tone all the small and large muscle fibers along the spine, including the rhomboid and mid-trapezius muscles of the upper back. Building tone in this way will help the spine and upper back maintain upright posture. (For Versions A and B, refer to Progressive Spinal Extensions, Pose 10, page 82.) Remember to choose only one of the versions of Locust pose presented here each time you practice that match your current needs and abilities.

CAUTION: If your low back begins to hurt in any of the variations offered here—STOP. Re-assess your pose to see if your tailbone is deep enough in and your spine as extended as long as possible. Alternately, return to the Locust pose Version A on a bolster offered in the Basic Low Back Sequence Pose 10 on page 26.

Version C–Alternate arm and leg lift

➤**1.** Lie on your belly, with your hips on a folded blanket. ➤**2.** Place your chin or forehead on the floor and extend your arms alongside your head. ➤**3.** Lift your inner legs up off the floor as you press your sacrum deeply down to lengthen your low back. Keep your feet on the floor. ➤**4.** Lift one leg and the opposite arm no more than 4 inches off the floor. ➤**5.** Hold for 3–5 breaths, release the arm and leg, and repeat with the other leg and opposite arm. ➤**6.** Repeat both diagonals a second time.

CAUTION: If you have trouble stabilizing your low back while pressing your sacrum in, move your hips back on the blanket so that the pubic bone is slightly off the blanket and the belly is more on it. You might also add an additional blanket.

Hint: Again less is more. Lift a minimal amount, but reach out through the raised arm and leg, while pressing your sacrum into the floor.

Pose 14 continued next page

Version D–Hands beside the chest

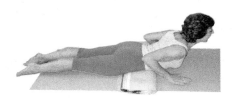

➤**1.** Lie on your belly, with your hips on a folded blanket, and place your hands beside your chest, palms down. ➤**2.** Lift your inner legs up off the floor as you press your sacrum deeply down to lengthen your low back. Keep your feet on the floor. ➤**3.** Roll your shoulders back and lift your chest, keeping your bottom front ribs down. ➤**4.** Draw the elbows back toward your feet as you press the bottom edge of the shoulder blades forward. ➤**5.** Lift your hands 1 inch off the floor and hold for 3–5 breaths. ➤**6.** Rest and repeat 3 times.

Hint: Elongate your spine by walking your bottom front ribs forward, and then roll your shoulders back and lift your chest.

Inner Action: Roll your little toe onto the floor to help you lift your inner thighs, while you take your sacrum and tailbone deep in to counterbalance your chest.

Version E–Arms extending back

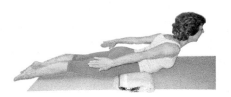

➤**1.** Repeat steps 1–4 from Version D above. ➤**2.** Extend your arms and hands back toward your feet with the palms facing in. ➤**3.** Keep your feet on the floor and your tailbone deep. ➤**4.** Hold for 3–5 breaths. Release and then repeat 2 times.

Hint: Maintain spinal length by moving your breastbone forward as you reach your hands and feet back.

CAUTION: Practice Version D until you have a clear sense of how to pin your shoulder blades to your back ribs, and keep the upper arm rolling back, before you reach back with your arms and hands.

Version F–Arms out to the side—Flying!

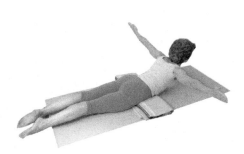

➤**1.** Repeat steps 1–4 from Version D above. ➤**2.** Lift your hands and slowly extend your arms out to the sides. ➤**3.** Face the palms forward, with the thumbs turned up. ➤**4.** Draw your inner shoulder blades down toward your waist as you turn your palms further up. ➤**5.** Then make the effort to lift your thumbs and arms skyward. ➤**6.** Hold for 3–5 breaths. Release, rest, and repeat once.

Hint 1: Keep the pelvis and thighs active to counterbalance the weight of the chest and arms.

Hint 2: Check to see that your arms are out to the side at the same height by turning your head slightly to see your thumbs.

CAUTION: This is the most challenging of the four arm positions offered in this book. Please be mindful to build up to this pose gradually.

POSE 15. **SIDEWAYS PLANK / VASISTHASANA**

Sideways Plank is a challenging pose that replaces the Lateral Leg Lift from the Basic Low Back Sequence. It will build tone in the side body, creating stability for the low back and hips, as well as strengthen the shoulder girdle. Begin practicing with your hand on a chair until you can easily hold your spine in a straight line, and then move the elbow or hand to the floor. Some students will prefer one version of the pose over the other—your choice.

Version A-Hand on a chair

➤**1.** Place all four chair legs on a sticky mat, or place the chair against a wall for safety. ➤**2.** Place your hand in the center of the chair, fingers pointing straight back. ➤**3.** Roll your right shoulder back and pin your shoulder blade to your back ribs. ➤**4.** Draw your armpit away from your arm so your ribs are lifting sideways away from the chair. ➤**5.** Step out with your right leg until your right side body is straight. ➤**6.** Place your left foot on top of your right, or allow it to remain on the floor just behind. ➤**7.** Keep your hips lifting and your shoulders rolled back. ➤**8.** Lift the back ribs and the front ribs equally away from the chair. Gaze straight ahead or at your top hand. ➤**9.** Hold for 3–5 breaths. Change sides.

Hint: Place your left foot slightly in back of your right ankle for balance.

Inner Action: Firm your legs. Lift the bottom of your belly in and up toward your chest and extend out the crown of your head.

CAUTION: Placement of the hand in relationship to your shoulder is important for the health of your wrist. When your hips are lifted, your shoulder should land no more than 1 inch or 2 behind the wrist so you can easily press the fingers of the hand down to create an even lift on the back of your wrist.

Version B-Elbow on the floor

➤**1.** Sitting sideways on the floor, place your elbow beneath your shoulder. ➤**2.** Roll your shoulder back and draw the shoulder blade toward your waist. ➤**3.** Extend your right leg and hook the sole of the foot on the floor. ➤**4.** With the left foot behind the right ankle, lift your hips up off the ground. ➤**5.** Lift the front and back of your hips evenly. ➤**6.** Concentrate on lifting your armpit chest away from the floor. ➤**7.** Hold for 3–5 breaths. Change sides.

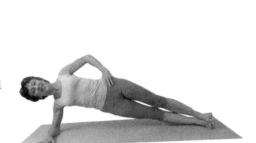

Hint: Do your best to place part of the sole of your foot on the mat to support the lift of your outer ankle and hips. Resting on your outer anklebone will increase the difficulty of the pose ten-fold.

CAUTION: If you feel strain in your shoulder joint or experience a feeling of collapsing, move back to Version A with the chair.

Version C-Hand on the floor

➤**1.** Begin by sitting sideways on the floor as in Version B. ➤**2.** Place your hand on the floor just ahead of your shoulder. ➤**3.** Roll your right shoulder back and pin your shoulder blade to your back ribs. ➤**4.** Draw your armpit away from your arm so your ribs are lifting sideways. ➤**5.** Place the left foot behind your right ankle. ➤**6.** Press the palm fully into the floor as you use your left foot to help lift your hips. ➤**7.** Gaze at your right hand and lift the back and front ribs equally. ➤**8.** When you find the balance, place the left foot on top of the right. (This is optional.) ➤**9.** Look straight ahead or slowly turn to look up. ➤**10.** Hold for 3–5 breaths. Change sides.

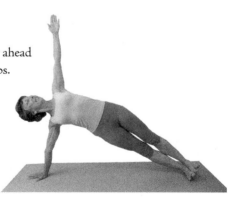

Hint: Position your bottom foot so that the outside edge of your sole is on the floor; this supports the lift of your hips slightly above the horizontal line.

CAUTION: As in Version A, placement of the hand in relationship to your shoulder is important for your wrist. When your hips are lifted, your shoulder should land no more than 1 inch or 2 behind the wrist so you can easily press the knuckles of the hand evenly down to create an even lift on the back of your wrist.

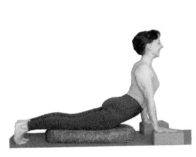

POSE 16. **REVERSE PLANK / PURVOTTANASANA**

Choose Version A with the hands on a chair, or for the more advanced practitioner, Version B with the hands on blocks on the floor. (For more details, refer to Progressive Spinal Extensions, Pose 7, page 80.)

➤**1.** Place your hands just behind your hips, either on the chair seat or on blocks on the floor. ➤**2.** Roll your shoulders back to pin your shoulders blades to your back ribs and lift your chest strongly up. ➤**3.** Exhale lift your hips. ➤**4.** Keep your knees bent and gaze forward. ➤**5.** Hold for 3–5 breaths and repeat 3 times.

Inner Action: Press the hands down and lift the front of your arm and chest up any amount.

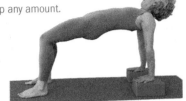

Note: When the muscles of the front of your arm and chest offer great resistance, try pulsing in and out of the pose on an exhale. After 3 or 4 rounds of working in this way, hold the pose for 3–5 breaths. Take your head back when possible without discomfort.

POSE 17. **UPWARD FACING DOG POSE / URDHVA MUKHA SVANASANA**

(For more details, see Progressive Spinal Extensions, Pose 8, page 81.)

Version A

➤**1.** Lie face down with the front edge of the bolster across the bottom of your belly and the blocks placed beside your waist. ➤**2.** Curl your toes under and firm your thighs by straightening your knees. ➤**3.** Keeping the knees firm, press your tail down into the bolster. ➤**4.** Inhale and roll your shoulders back and draw your breastbone forward and up as you did in the door chest hang. ➤**5.** Straighten your arms as much as possible.

Remember: Lengthen your front spine from the bottom of the belly to the bottom tip of the breastbone, and then curl the upper chest back. Check to see if your wrists are directly under your shoulders.

Inner Action: Continue to reach back through your heels and ground down through your tailbone as you straighten your arms as much as possible, lifting your chest.

Version B

➤**1.** Place your hands just in front of your hips on the chair seat, fingers pointing out. ➤**2.** Roll your chest open from front to back by first bending your elbows, and then straightening your arms. ➤**3.** Lift the bottom of your belly in and up toward your chest as you extend back through your legs. ➤**4.** Hold for 3–5 breaths. Repeat.

Remember: As you press your thighs back and up, squeeze your sacrum deep in and connect to the lift of your chest.

Hint: When practicing with your hands on a chair, draw back into down dog, in between attempts at up dog, to release any tension in your spine as a counter-balancing pose helping you create optimal length in your spine.

Inner Action: Squeeze the point of the elbow forward and lift up from the inner elbow to the front shoulder. Finish the loop, drawing the top of the back arm down toward the point of the elbow, to feel your chest curl further.

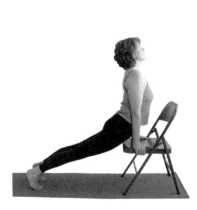

POSE 18. **SIDEWAYS CHAIR TWIST / BHARADVAJASANA**

(For more details, refer to Basic Neck and Shoulder Sequence, Pose 11, page 32.)

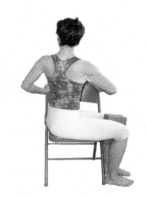

➤**1.** Sit sideways in a chair with a block between your knees. ➤**2.** Adjust the chair to match your height by placing a folded blanket under your hips until your thighs are parallel to the floor. ➤**3.** Lift your front spine to create length, and then turn toward the chair back. ➤**4.** On the exhalation, deflate your lower belly and turn. ➤**5.** Hold for 3–5 breaths. Change sides.

Remember: This twisting pose here acts as a counterbalancing pose to release the spinal muscles from any tension built from the work of weight bearing.

Inner Action: Progress up the spine one section at a time, turning with each exhale, and keeping your ribs level.

POSE 19. **SUPPORTED PELVIC LIFT / SETU BANDHA SARVANGASANA**

Version C–Block under sacrum

(For more details, see Progressive Spinal Extensions, Pose 2, page 77.)

The intention of practicing this version of the pose here is to relax the whole body by using the support of the block and breathing in a deep and relaxed pattern to release the work of the spine. To relax fully make your exhalations longer than your inhalations.

Place the block sideways under your mid-sacrum for stability and rest. The photo shows the block narrow under the mid-sacrum, which is a more active version suitable for the spinal extension practice. If your hips feel at all unstable, stay with the sideways block.

➤**1.** Lift your hips high enough to place the block under your mid-sacrum. ➤**2.** Without lifting your hips off the block, curl your tail between the legs as you draw the skin from behind your pubic bone in and up toward your chest to open the psoas and front hip. ➤**3.** Turn your upper arm and shoulders under, toward your spine. Press your arms down lightly to lift your chest.
➤**4.** Continue to raise your breastbone toward your chin and soften your front throat.
➤**5.** Hold for 5–7 breaths.

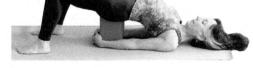

Inner Action: Be sure to keep lifting your breastbone toward your chin to elongate your organs and traction the spine to relieve any pinching in the joints. Take slow deep breaths.

CAUTION: If your low back pinches, move the block closer to your tailbone to lengthen your lumbar curve.

POSE 20. **SUPINE BOUND ANGLE ROCK / SUPTA BADDHA KONASANA**

This lovely pose is placed here as a final counterbalancing to release the low back before relaxation.

After completing the pose, simply stretch out flat on the floor for a simple Corpse Pose. (For more details, see Alternate Low Back Sequence, Pose 12, page 41.)

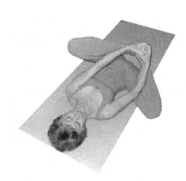

➤**1.** Place the soles of your feet together and hold either your ankles or your feet. ➤**2.** Draw your feet toward your chest and keep your knees wide. ➤**3.** Rock gently side to side, bringing each knee to touch the floor. ➤**4.** Rock back and forth 4–5 times.

Inner Action: Lengthen the back of your neck and soften your jaw, allowing your head to naturally follow your knees as they rock.

Leg Toning Sequence

As you move forward building your spinal health, it's important to address the muscle tone of your legs. I hope you've come to recognize and experience through the previous sequences how the legs extend the spine—that the reaching out of our legs activates the energy flow to our spines, allowing us to create the length and space so essential to finding pain relief.

Now it's time to combine much of what you've already learned in order to establish greater tone and integration of the legs with the spine. In this way, you'll continue to build self-confidence and self-reliance. The practice of yoga offers many different standing poses that tone the legs. Some of those poses are not suitable for certain back conditions; therefore, in consideration of everyone's safety, I've added only three additional poses to balance the strength of this sequence; Sideways Lunge, Split Leg Forward Fold, and Straddle Forward Fold. Because you're now familiar with the other poses, I am presenting them here with a photo, brief instructions, and the reference to the pages on which you can find more information.

This sequence contains 17 poses that will initially require 45–60 minutes to complete.

POSE 1. **BASIC LYING TWIST / JATHARA PARIVARTANASANA**

(For more information, see Pose 6 in the Abdominal Progressions for Back Care, page 36.)
Repetitions warm the body, tone the transverse and oblique abdominals, and release tension in the spine.

➤**1.** Be sure to fully extend your arms when you draw the knees toward your chest. ➤**2.** As you exhale, roll over your hip to twist your knees to the right, stop half way or continue to 6–10 inches away from the floor. ➤**3.** Again exhale, drop the lower belly in, and turn your bottom ribs from the center of your clock face to the left. ➤**4.** Use your exhale to move you in and out of the pose. ➤**5.** Hold 1–2 breaths, change sides, and repeat 3–5 times.

Remember: Gradually take your knees closer to the floor while keeping your opposite ribs down.

Hint: Be certain the knees are closer to your chest than your navel to elongate and release the spine.

Inner Action: Mentally connect and draw from the right groin to the left bottom ribs to turn the upper belly toward the floor.

POSE 2. **TRACTION TWIST / SUPTA MATSYANGASANA**

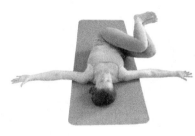

(See Pose 1 in the Basic Low Back Sequence, page 23, for more details.)
This simple pose does a great job of opening the psoas muscle, and also tractions the lumbar spine one side at a time.

➤**1.** Lie on your back, step your feet to the sides of your mat, and drop both knees to the left. ➤**2.** Extend out from the right hip to the right knee. ➤**3.** Curl your tail toward your pubic bone, as you draw the bottom of the belly in and up.

Hint: Curl your tail so much that the bottom of your belly becomes hollow and your organs release and drop in toward your spine.

CAUTION: Flex your feet to protect your knee. Use a block under the knee as necessary for support.

POSE 3. **ALTERNATING KNEE CURL-UPS /APANASANA VARIATION**

(See Pose 3 in Progressive Abdominal Toning, page 34, for more details.)
Here you're toning the transverse abdominus, psoas, and oblique abdominal muscles, engaging their support. You may choose to do one or both of the following variations:

Version A

➤**1.** Keep your left foot on the floor and hold onto your right kneecap. ➤**2.** Press your right knee out to arm's length to create resistance as you draw the center of your clock face in and up. ➤**3.** Curl the head and chest up toward the right knee, keeping the knee stationary. ➤**4.** Draw the elbows out and up as the inner shoulders draw down. ➤**5.** Hold for 3–5 breaths. Change sides. Repeat 3 times.

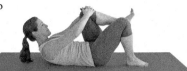

Version B

➤**1.** Repeat steps 1–4 from Version A. ➤**2.** Extend the left leg straight up, and lower it with an exhale, until your foot is 4–10 inches off the floor. ➤**3.** Hold for 3–5 breaths. Change sides. Repeat 3 times.

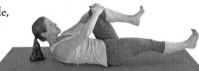

Hint: Be certain to remain balanced on the center of your clock face as well as drawing in and up.

POSE 4. **YOGI CURL-UPS**

(Refer to Pose 12 in the Basic Low Back Sequence, page 27, for more details.)
This familiar pose tones the upper abdominal muscles and the long fibers of the psoas without engaging the lower fibers of the illio-psoas muscles. Start by doing Version B, and then practice Version C.

Version B

➤**1.** Begin *lying* on your back with your knees bent and feet on the floor. Or choose to place your feet on a wall or chair, with your legs at right angles for more release in the low back. ➤**2.** Cross your arms behind your head for additional neck support, with each hand touching the opposite shoulder. ➤**3.** Curl up one third of the way. Keep your chin neutral, with the eyes gazing at your knees. ➤**4.** Hold the position for 3–5 breaths.

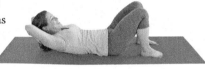

Version C

➤**5.** Again, curl-up one third of the way. ➤**6.** Add a twist by bringing the left shoulder toward your right knee, then your right shoulder toward the left knee. ➤**7.** Hold for 3–5 breaths. Observe which side seems weak, and hold that position longer.

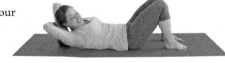

Hint: Keep your inner groin soft, feet grounded. Breathe by expanding your side ribs.

POSE 5. **YOGA LEG LIFTS / URDHVA PRASARITA PADASANA**

(Refer to Pose 5 in Progressive Abdominal Toning on page 35 for more details.)
There are three possible methods for doing this pose. Choose the one that suits your current abilities, being certain to keep your clock face down because the low back is the most secure in that position. For this sequence I'm recommending Version A as it builds tone in the legs and is the most secure version for the lower back.

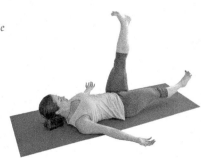

Version A

➤**1.** Lie on your back with your arms extended out to the side. ➤**2.** Bring your knees to your chest and extend both legs up. ➤**3.** Lift the head for additional safety and support, and gaze toward your knees. ➤**4.** Lower one leg at a time until it's 4–10 inches off the floor. ➤**5.** Exhale to lower the leg; inhale to lift the leg back up. ➤**6.** Repeat for 3 rounds.

Hint: Control your legs from the center of your clock face, pulling it strongly in and up toward your chest as you exhale. Strongly extend both knees.

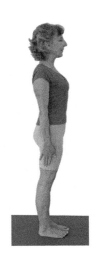

POSE 6. **STAND TALL / TADASANA**

(Refer to the Basic Low Back Sequence on page 25 for more information.)
Standing Tall is a foundational asana in yoga because its key aspects are reflected in many other poses, especially the standing poses being presented in this sequence.

➤**1.** Stand with a block between your feet so both the big toe mound and inner heel make contact.
➤**2.** To lift the inner arch of the foot, bring the inner knee joints forward to face each other, while turning your outer top shins back. ➤**3.** Now squeeze the block with your big toe mound to move the inner groin back to the center of the pelvic floor. ➤**4.** Reach your heels into the floor as you lift the bottom of your belly up. ➤**5-.** Lift your inner body up from your inner leg to your pelvic floor, and from the pelvic floor up to your chest. ➤**6.** Roll the shoulders back and down as you lift the center of your chest high.
➤**7.** Now hug the block with your inner heel to wrap the outer shin and thigh back.

Hint: Be certain to take your top thighs back far enough for your pelvic floor to be in line with the crown of your head. Extend up through your crown.

POSE 7. **SIDEWAYS LUNGE/ VIRABHADRASANA II**

This pose offers horizontal opening to the pelvis and lengthens the inner legs, or adductors. When done correctly, the pose also strengthens the buttock muscles and pelvic floor.

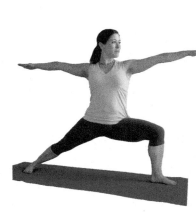

➤**1.** Begin by Standing Tall, and then take your feet 3.5–4 feet apart—ideally one leg- length apart.
➤**2.** Turn your right foot in halfway; allow your kneecap and hips to face in the same direction.
➤**3.** Turn your left foot and leg out 90 degrees. ➤**4.** Lift the bottom of your belly as you draw the top of your buttocks toward the floor. ➤**5.** With your hands on your hips, press down to lift your chest and ribs up. ➤**6.** Turn your ribs to face forward as you raise your arms to the sides. ➤**7.** Lift your left hip up and lower your right hip until your pelvic floor is parallel to the earth. ➤**8.** With an exhale, press down into the right heel as you bend your front knee, pointing it toward your second toe. ➤**9.** Extend from the left inner groin toward your knee, and then turn the skin of the knee from inside out. ➤**10.** Next draw the skin from your outer left knee toward your buttocks to coil your left hip into its socket.
➤**11.** Reach into your back leg and arm and hold for 5–7 breaths. Change sides.

Hint: Once you're in the pose, continue to coil your left hip in as you turn your left knee and right hipbone away from each other to open horizontally and move your hips closer to parallel.

CAUTION 1: DO NOT square your hips to the side of your mat. Attempting to square your hips is likely to create distress in your hip, sacral, and knee joints.

CAUTION 2: It's important to keep 3:00 and 9:00 on the same line, parallel to the floor, to avoid pinching the tube of the lumbar spine. This is especially important if you're healing from a low back disc injury, or if you've lost disc space in the lumbar area. If you feel any cramping or nerve pinching in your legs, modify, avoid the pose, or seek professional help.

POSE 8. **STANDING LUNGE / VIRABHADRASANA I**

(Refer to Pose 5, Progressive Spinal Extensions, on page 79 for more details).
To work your legs well, practice one of the variations of the classical pose presented here.

Version A

This version of placing the foot on a chair is recommended for very stiff bodies, as well as for situations where there maybe a bulging disc. Raising the knee helps keep the pelvis from collapsing forward, thus protecting the lower back. Place the chair against the wall or place all four legs on a sticky mat to prevent the chair from slipping.

➤**1.** Place your left foot on the seat of the chair. ➤**2.** Root down into the outer rear heel of the standing leg as you lift from the back of the knee toward your buttock to draw the top thigh further back. ➤**3.** Now draw the top of your buttocks down and lift the bottom of the belly without bending the back knee. ➤**4.** Inhale and raise your arms overhead. ➤**5.** Exhale and lift the palms of your hands away from your hips to lengthen your spine. ➤**6.** With your next exhalation, draw the bottom of your belly in and up as you bend the front knee any amount. ➤**7.** Continue extending as you hold the pose for 3 breaths.

Hint: If the buttock of your back leg is soft, then root into the rear heel, lift up from the back of the knee and pull the top of your buttocks down and lift the bottom of your belly until you engage the buttock muscles.

Inner Action: As you root down through the outer rear heel, lift up the inner leg into and through the pelvic floor, along the inner spine, and connect to the lift of the chest.

Remember: Keep your front ribs drawn down and balanced over your pelvis so your clock face is flat. When shoulder flexibility is limited you will need to lower your arms to do so.

Version C

The version with the rear heel up on the wall is a good alternative for extending the back leg and spine completely when the calf muscles are short, if there's been injury to the knee or ankle, or if the knee or ankle is tender in any way. Plus, in this version, it's easier to keep your clock face level and lifted, protecting your lower back.

➤**1.** Place your right heel up the wall at a 45-degree angle. ➤**2.** Turn you hips to face forward and step your left foot out as far as possible keeping your hips square. ➤**3.** Use your hands on your hips to press down as you lift the bottom of your belly in and up to raise your chest. ➤**4.** As you exhale bend your front knee any amount. ➤**5.** Continue to extend the inner rear heel into the wall as you lift from your pelvic floor to your chest. ➤**6.** Pause on the inhale, extend the leg, and lift your spine with each exhalation. ➤**7.** Hold for 3–5 breaths.

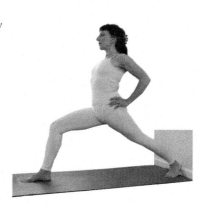

Hint: As you lift the bottom of the belly, the rear knee will want to bend. Maintain the extension of the rear knee by exaggerating the connection of that heel to the wall as you slowly bend the front knee any amount.

Hint 2: You can balance your clock face from the front or back of your pelvis—either by scooping the bottom of the bent knee buttock and tailbone forward, or by lifting the front hip bones evenly. Try both to see which one is most helpful to you.

Inner Action: As you lift the bottom of your belly in and up, squeeze your outer left hip in toward your midline just enough to balance over your pelvic floor (i.e., 3:00 and 9:00) so the buttock muscles of the rear leg become active.

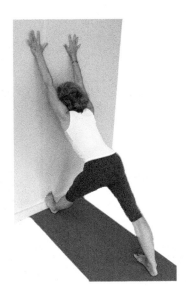

POSE 9. **SPLIT LEG FORWARD FOLD / PARSVOTTANASANA**

To maintain length in the spine while strengthening the legs, I offer you this variation of a forward fold. The intent is to stretch the hamstrings in a weight-bearing pose, as well as tone the opposite or quadricep muscles. Practice both versions.

Version A–Hands on the wall

➤**1.** Facing the wall, place the ball of the right foot on the wall so your foot is at a 45-degree angle. ➤**2.** Step your left foot back one leg length or less, depending on your flexibility, with the foot turned slightly out. ➤**3.** Walk your hands up the wall and position your arms as you would for Downward Facing Dog pose. ➤**4.** Square your hips to the wall, and then exhale and press your top thighs back as far as possible to hinge at your hip joint. ➤**5.** Pull up on your kneecaps to lift the quadricep muscles. ➤**6.** Sharpen the point of your sits bones. ➤**7.** Hold for 3–5 breaths. Change sides.

Hint 1: Think of rooting your heels deeper into the floor, and then pull up from the head of your calf muscles toward your sits bones to lengthen your hamstrings.

Hint 2: Micro-bend your front knee to lift the kneecap and firm your quadriceps.

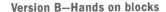

Version B—Hands on blocks

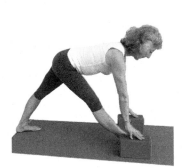

➤**1.** In this version, place your right heel against the baseboard at the wall, with the toes turned out 25 degrees. ➤**2.** Step your left foot forward one leg length and micro bend your knee to point the knee cap toward the second and third toe. ➤**3.** Place your hands on your hips to level the balance of your clock face. ➤**4.** Press your heels into the floor and lift the bottom of your belly strongly up. ➤**5.** As you exhale, hinge at your hips to send your sits bones back and extend your chest forward. ➤**6.** Keeping your spine extended, place your hands on the blocks. ➤**7.** With an exhale, continue to firm your knee caps by lifting from the head of the calf to the sits bones. ➤**8.** Hold for 3–5 breaths. Change sides.

Hint: Remember to align the front knee with the center of the foot. Move the inner knee forward and turn the outer top shin back to balance and lift the inner arch. Then, tuck the outer top hip in toward the tailbone to maintain the stability of your hips, keeping your clock face parallel to the floor.

Note: The blocks have three heights. For limited flexibility stack two blocks under each hand or place your hands on a chair.

POSE 10. **STANDING SCISSOR TWIST / PARSVA HASTA PADASANA**

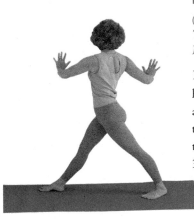

(For more details, see Pose 7 in Progressive Twists, page 65.)
This pose requires strong muscular action in the legs to keep the rear heel rooted with the belly and spine lifting. It also extends the front thigh, psoas muscle, and front spine as one unit to decompress the spine.

➤**1.** When you've moved into your triangle position with your legs, actively press down into the rear heel as you extend from the back of your rear knee up toward your buttock. ➤**2.** Move your tail forward and lift the skin of your pubis in and up to elongate your clock face. ➤**3.** Exhale and turn your navel toward the wall as far as possible, keeping the back heel rooting down. ➤**4.** Use the wall for leverage to help turn your chest. ➤**5.** Keep your nose centered over your breastbone as you turn. ➤**6.** Hold for 3–5 breaths and repeat. Change sides.

Hint: For more stability, stand closer to the wall. Remember less is more—be happy with small movements. Pull up on the skin of your lower belly as you root your heels down.

POSE 11. **STANDING CHAIR TWIST / MARICHYASANA III**

(See Pose 16, Alternate Low Back Sequence, page 43, for more information.).
This pose will relieve tension along the spine by stretching the small muscles that connect one vertebra to another, as well as build tone in the legs to help you gain length in your spine.

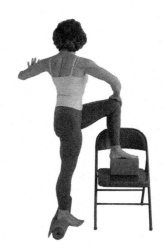

➤**1.** Stand beside and close to the chair, with your heels optionally elevated on a mat roll. ➤**2.** Place the foot that is closest to the wall on the block on the chair. ➤**3.** Stand in the back of your leg by aligning the center of your hip with your knee and ankle. ➤**4.** Lift your chest and spine from the center of your clock face, and then twist toward the wall. ➤**5.** With your opposite hand, hold the bent knee stationary and steady as you turn. ➤**6.** Imagine a line from your inner ankle to the crown of your head, and turn your spine around that line, beginning with the center of your clock face. ➤**7.** Hold for 3–5 breaths. Repeat each side twice.

Hint: If your low back is very tender, be sure to use a mat roll under the standing heel to further lift and decompress your spine.

Hint 2: Think about the tube of the leg and move the contents of the leg away from the skin and into the center of the 'tube'.

POSE 12. **STANDING HAND TO FOOT POSE / UTTHITA HASTA PADANGUSTHASANA**

(Refer to Pose 17 in the Alternate Low Back Sequence on page 44 for more information.)
This pose creates length in the legs and spine, as well as builds strength in the legs and pelvic ring.

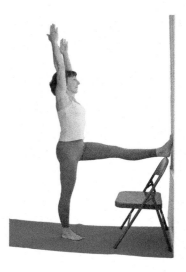

➤**1.** Place your left heel on the back of the chair, toes touching the wall. ➤**2.** Align your standing leg from the inner ankle to the center knee to the inner groin. ➤**3.** Move your inner groins back to the center of your pelvic floor, and then lift the bottom of the belly and draw the top buttocks down. ➤**4.** Squeeze in on the outside thigh of your standing leg to help stabilize the hips. ➤**5.** Then lift up through the inner leg and midline of your body to the crown of your head. ➤**6.** Extend from the back of both knees toward the buttocks to straighten your knees. ➤**7.** Raise your arms above your head and lift your palms up from the sides of your hips to extend your spine further. ➤**8.** Balance the clock face of your pelvis so the left and right hipbones are level. ➤**9.** Hold for 3–5 breaths. Repeat each side twice.

Hint 1: Test the water to determine at what height you will need to place the top foot so you can straighten both knees. Use a block on the chair seat to lower the leg as necessary to match your hamstring length. The block has three heights to choose from—low, medium, and tall.

Hint 2: Hug your sits bones in toward your tailbone to create more stability in your hips.

Hint 3: Be mindful of your standing leg and micro-bend the knee to avoid hyperextension of the knee. The alignment of the leg will give you more lift in your spine. Again, think to move the contents of the tube to its center.

POSE 13. **STANDING HAND TO FOOT AND TWIST / PARIVRTTA HASTA PADANGUSTHASANA**

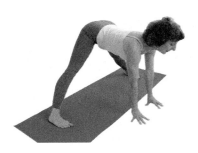

(Refer to Pose 10 in Progressive Twists on page 66 for more details.) This pose opens the outer leg, improving mobility in your hips while toning the legs. The pose also aligns the spine by releasing tension as well as building strength.

➤**1.** Begin as you did in the previous pose, be sure to re-create the alignment of the standing leg and straighten both legs. ➤**2.** Raise your arms above your head and lift your spine. ➤**3.** Stabilize your hips by lifting strongly through the inner standing leg and pelvic floor before turning. ➤**4.** Turn from your navel and bottom ribs any amount toward the top leg, and place your opposite hand outside the knee. ➤**5.** Press the back of the hand into the knee and continue to turn with your exhalation. ➤**6.** Balance in the center of your standing leg and level your hips as much as possible by drawing your sits bones toward each other. ➤**7.** Hold for 3–5 breaths. Repeat each side twice.

Hint: To avoid over extending the shoulder of the extended arm, press your palm into an imaginary glass wall as you twist your chest toward the arm. The arm will always be in full view.

POSE 14. **STRADDLE FORWARD FOLD CONCAVE / PRASARITA PADOTTANASANA**

This is one of the most stable poses for the hips and low back when bending forward. Widening the legs with this pose opens the pelvic floor, creating horizontal space and release for the spine to fully extend.

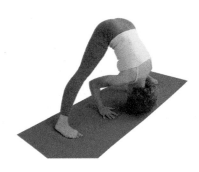

➤**1.** Standing in the center of your mat step, your feet 3.5–4.5 feet apart. This is a wide stance. ➤**2.** Pivot on your heels and turn your toes in 10-15 degrees so the heels are wider apart and you're slightly pigeon-toed. ➤**3.** Place your hands on your hips to balance and level your clock face. ➤**4.** Press your heels into the floor and lift your knees, thigh muscles, and the bottom of your belly strongly up. ➤**5.** As you exhale, hinge at your hips to send your sits bones back, and extend your chest forward. ➤**6.** Keeping your spine extended, place your hands on the floor or blocks. ➤**7.** Inhale and move your breastbone forward and up as you draw your shoulder blades toward your waist, arching your upper back slightly. ➤**8.** Exhale and lift from the head of the calf to the sits bones to open and move your top thighs back any amount. ➤**9.** Hold for 3–5 breaths.

Hint 1: Avoid hyper-extending your knees by shifting your weight slightly forward and micro bending your knees before lifting the head of the calf up.

Hint 2: Coming out of a pose is as important as going in. Lift your head and chest, hands to your hips, and then pull your tail down and your heels in toward the center to stand up.

CAUTION: It's important to keep your spine extended. Adjust the height of the blocks to allow you to do so. If your hamstrings are very short, you may need to place your hands on the seat of a chair.

POSE 15. **STRADDLE FORWARD FOLD ROUNDED BACK/ PRASARITA PADOTTANASANA**

A continuation of the previous pose, this position completes the extension and release of the spine, as well as lengthens the hamstring muscles fully.

➤**1.** Begin in the flat back position with the hands on the blocks as above. ➤**2.** Exhale and fold forward, hinging at the top thighs, and walk your hands back, keeping your front spine long. ➤**3.** Release your head down. ➤**4.** Shift your weight forward until you feel your heels become light, and then lift your toes. This will unlock your knee, ground your heels, and allow your hamstrings to stretch. ➤**5.** Open from the outer back knees up to your sits bones, and then anchor the outside edge of your foot. ➤**6.** Draw the outer shin and outer top thigh back to elongate your lower belly. ➤**7.** Hold for 3–5 breaths. Come out of the pose the same way you went in.

Hint: As you shift your weight forward, lift your shoulders up toward your waist to keep your chest from collapsing into your neck.

CAUTION: in this version the head will not touch the floor in order to create more length in the spine.

POSE 16. **PELVIC LIFTS / SETU BANDHA SARVANGASANA**

(For more information, refer Pose 10 in the Alternate Low Back Sequence, page 40.)
Stabilize your hips with this pose, which lengthens the quadricep muscles, tones the gluteal muscles, and integrates the psoas muscles on both sides. To encourage optimal release of the psoas muscles to balance this sequence, please lift your hips only halfway up to allow the psoas to hang like a hammock holding your internal organs. Then progress into the full pose.

➤**1.** Press up into the pose halfway, being sure to curl your tail and slide your knees forward to lift your hips. ➤**2.** After a couple of breaths, press your heels down to lift your hips higher. ➤**3.** Turn the upper arms out and under your chest, shoulders blades moving toward the spine. ➤**4.** Press your arms down to raise your breastbone toward your chin in order to elongate your spine and protect your lower back. ➤**5.** Repeat the lift 3 times, holding for 5–7 breaths.

Version A

Begin by holding a block between your knees to tone the inner thighs and release the outer hips and low back as you lift. This is an excellent version for a person with very strong hip flexors.

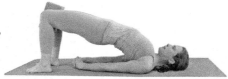

Version B

Place a belt loop approximately 4–6 inches above your knees. As you lift, press out into the belt to activate and tone the gluteal muscles, an excellent choice for persons who experience low back weakness or sacroiliac instability.

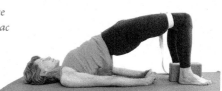

Hint: Peel the spine up off the floor, extending the knees slightly forward. Roll down slowly, with the back of the waist touching before the hips. Moving in this way will encourage the release, integration, and balance of the psoas muscles.

POSE 17. **CORPSE POSE / SAVASANA**

As always, time spent at rest is vital to the restoration of our nerves and for the integration of all parts of ourselves. Choose any version of Corpse Pose—A, B, C—from the Basic Low Back and the Basic Neck and Shoulder Sequences on pages 27 and 32. Or use the full Supported Pelvic Lift described here in place of the classic savasana. Give yourself 5 minutes to be still, observe, and feel the effect of your practice.

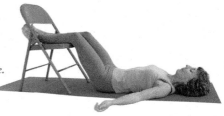

SUPPORTED PELVIC LIFT / SETU BHANDA SARVANGASANA

(For a full description of this pose, see Pose 2, in the Six Basic Restorative Poses on page 48.)
Everyone can do this pose, as it's a foundational pose for most therapeutic yoga practices. With the head and neck positioned below the heart, this pose is a mild inversion, and all the benefits of an inversion apply. It provides a very deep and quick recovery from the fatigue of the Leg Toning Sequence.

➤**1.** Begin with two bolsters placed end-to-end, or 4 lengthwise folded blankets in two stacks, placed end-to-end. ➤**2.** Sit with your hips on the bolster or blankets, knees bent. ➤**3.** Lift your hips and move the flesh of your buttocks toward your feet. ➤**4.** Lie back on the bolster or blankets with the bottom edge of your shoulder blades in contact, i.e., hooked on the edge of the support. ➤**5.** Your shoulders will not be touching the floor; however, the back of your neck will feel long. ➤**6.** Straighten your legs and relax your arms out to the sides. ➤**7.** Stay in this position for 7 or more minutes. ➤**8.** To come out, bend your knees and roll to your right side.

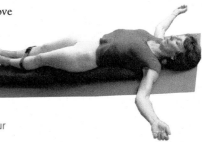

Hint: You may find it more relaxing to place a belt around your thighs or calves, as shown in the photo, to hold your legs so you can let go completely.

Self-Applied Back Care Quick Review: Part 2

1. *When a person with back pain begins a yoga practice, what is the appropriate treatment plan?* Always create length and space in the muscles and joints before you begin to strengthen muscles. If you begin to feel discomfort or negative pain in your injured area, go back to basic poses to find relief.

2. *Name the 3 twists that are best for first-aid relief for back pain.* Traction Twist, Standing Chair Twist, and Prone Twist on a Bolster.

3. *Name 3 other reliable twists that you have found helpful for acute back pain.* Review the twists in the Progressive Twists for Back Care on page 63. Begin with Pose 2–Basic Lying Twist, Pose 3–Yogi Curl Ups with a Twist, Pose 5–Sideways Chair Twist, and Pose 6–Open Chair Twist. These are all excellent foundational twists.

4. *Explain why the Hip Sequence is important to spinal health and function?* This sequence offers the opportunity to create muscular balance in the hip joints. Balanced mobility helps us in several ways–by creating a more even gate, an extended stride, and a more even weight distribution when we're standing. When the tubes of the legs are aligned with the center of the pelvic floor underneath us, there is less stress and more support for our spines, and thus our ability to maintain length.

5. *Name 3 ways to practice the Standing Lunge / Virabhadrasana I and cite the benefit of each.*

   1. With the front foot on a chair seat. By raising the foot like this, the low back is protected from collapsing. This is an excellent choice when there is a herniated disc, or if the muscles of the legs are overly muscular.

   2. With the front knee pressing a block into the wall. This version stabilizes the pelvis and gives resistance in order to lift and tone the bottom of the belly, while also lengthening the psoas muscles.

   3. With the rear heel up on the wall. This version extends the back leg and spine completely when the calf muscles are short, or the rear knee is tender, and/or recovering from an injury.

6. *Name 3 ways to practice Pelvic Lifts / Setu Bandha and cite the benefit of each.*

   1. Hold a block between the knees. This version overcomes tight quadricep muscles and keeps the knees running parallel, which helps avoid any low back pinching.

   2. Place a belt around both thighs 4–6 inches above the knees. This position helps to tone the buttock muscles and stabilize the sacroiliac joints.

   3. With a block under the mid-point of the sacrum. This version passively opens the hip flexors and allows a person to stay in the pose long enough for the muscles to let go. Remember the block has three heights.

7. *Which poses are helpful to lengthen the psoas muscles?* All the poses from Progressive Spinal Extensions on page 75 will do this, with the exception of Pose 9–Downward Facing Dog and Pose 11–Wide Leg Child's Pose, which are counterbalancing poses in which you fold forward.

8. *Which poses will tone the psoas muscles?* Any poses that tone the abdominal muscles will generally tone the psoas as well. See Progressive Abdominal Toning on page 33.

9. *Why is the balance of the psoas muscles important?* The psoas muscles are core muscles that support the front of the spine on the inside and create the curves of our spine. A short psoas pulls the pelvis forward, causing an excess lower back curve and loss of support. The shortening of the long and short fibers of the psoas tend to make the whole spine shorter. Lengthening the psoas muscles by extending the front body aids the human form in coming to its full upright posture.

10. *Rounded shoulders indicate an imbalance in which muscle groups? Which poses could you perform to rebalance?* The pectoralis muscles of the front chest are powerful and short, causing the mid-trapezius and rhomboid muscles between the shoulder blades to loose tone. The latissimus dorsi might also be short, pulling the front shoulders down. Practicing the Door Chest Hang (see page 32) consistently will help release and lengthen the front chest, while simultaneously toning the upper back muscles. Elbow on a Chair Seat from the Basic Neck and Shoulder Sequence (see page 31) stretches the latissimus dorsi. Other choices can be found in the Shoulder Release Sequence on page 70.

11. *If you experience numbness in your hands or arms when performing stretches to release tension in the shoulders, what is the best way to proceed?* Always back off 10 percent when it's unclear if the sensations are indicating positive or negative pain. As there is at times unavoidable nerve pinching in the arms and hands do to overly tight muscles tendons and fascia, don't push. Breathe deeply and go in and out of the pose for short timings. Be persistent yet patient.

12. *Describe the benefits of weight bearing and non-weight bearing poses.* Weight bearing poses create heat and strength in the muscles. Non-weight bearing poses create length and space and allow us to sensitively adjust our poses to release any pinching of the tubes.

part 3

Stabilizing the Pelvic Floor and Sacrum

Deepening your yoga practice will bring you in touch with the need for reciprocal muscular action to maintain and create stability in the pelvic floor and sacroiliac joints. This section addresses the four types of sacroiliac joint disturbances, teaches you how to evaluate your particular imbalance, and offers pose sequences to help you move toward stability and balance.

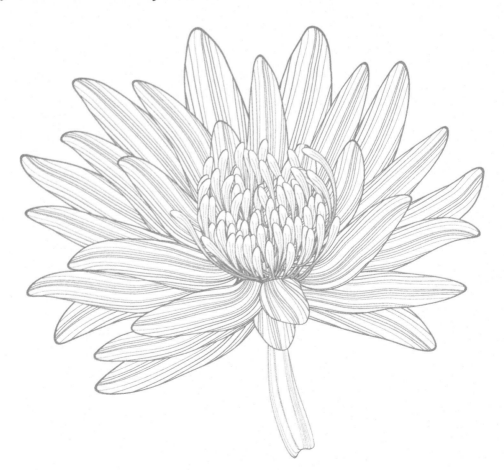

Pelvic Floor & Sacroiliac Joint Asymmetry

One of the real challenges in the practice and teaching of yoga is to understand the need for reciprocal muscular action to maintain, and/or create stability in the pelvic floor and sacroiliac joints (SI joints). Because the pelvic ring or bowl is the body's major weight-transmitting structure between the earth and the spine, disturbances here have the potential to throw off the whole structure, creating joint pain and dysfunction in the hips, knees, back, and shoulders. Learning how to balance the suppleness and strength of the pelvic floor and create stability in the SI joints are the focus of this section.

One of the first questions I ask a student who complains of back or hip pain is, "Did you ever fall on a hip or your tailbone?" The answer to this question is an important first step to help them identify their imbalance. Sacroiliac imbalance or derangement may also be a product of birthing a child, repetitive motion, such as driving a truck for 30 years, stress factors, or scoliosis i.e., curvatures of the spine.

Anatomically, the SI joints sit to the inside of the posterior hipbones and form the base of the spine. The sacrum belongs to the spine, even though it's attached to the hips at the SI joint. The SI joints can present in more than six different misalignment configurations as understood by physiatrists and chiropractors. That depth of understanding is beyond the scope of this book. However, the four types listed here refer to the relationships of the ligaments and muscles, simplifying the approach to a potentially confusing topic, and offering remedies to those who have these types of misalignments.

When the sacroiliac joint is causing pain, it's typically felt just off center to the left or the right in the dimple below the crest of the hipbone. The concentration of pain usually feels like the size of a quarter and can radiate from there. The pain may be felt in both sides and may also radiate through to the front of the groin, or create compression and pain in the lower lumbar vertebrae. As the piriformis muscle is one of the main stabilizers of the sacrum, a misalignment or derangement can cause the muscle to go into spasm and irritate the sciatic nerve. The secret to finding relief with yoga is to balance and tone the large and small muscles of the pelvis.

Four Types of Sacroiliac Joint Disturbance

There are four main types of imbalances that disturb the sacroiliac joints. The examination of these four types provides the basis for how to adjust our yoga practice for optimal results and pain relief.

Type 1. Both SI ligaments are loose and the muscles are loose. This often occurs in women after several pregnancies, in people who carry too much bodyweight without enough exercise, or when there is a genetic predisposition to loose ligaments. A person experiencing a Type 1 disturbance will often complain of pain over both sacroiliac joints and may walk with a vertical waddle. If Type 1 describes your situation, choose poses that tone the abdominals, hips, and legs, rather than stretches that may pull the SI joints out of alignment, resulting in a return to the pain loop. Poses recommended: Yogi Curl Ups, Alternating Knee Curl Ups, Basic Lying Twist (half way or less to tone the abdominals), Pelvic Lifts holding a block, and the Sacral Stabilization Sequence found on page 110. It's best to avoid twisting poses, with the exceptions of Basic Lying Twist, Sideways Chair Twist and Open Chair Twist on page 71.

Hint: If you suspect this condition, buy yourself a sacral belt to wear when lifting, vacuuming, or gardening. The belt with replace the lost tone in the muscles and ligaments, offering stability for the pelvis and spine. It's just another yoga prop—better safe than sorry.

Type 2. Both SI ligaments are tight and the muscles are loose. This occurs more typically in men, young or ageing, as well as some women. It can be recognized by an alteration in smooth walking with a horizontal wiggle, in which the hips look like they twist a bit with each step. This wiggle causes excessive movement and strain in L4/L5 and L5/S1. The quadriceps, hamstrings, and buttock muscles are usually loose, but they may also be tight. To address this imbalance, perform the Basic Low Back Sequence on page 23, the Alternate Low back Sequence on page 37, and the Leg Toning Sequence on page 94.

Type 3. Both SI ligaments and muscles are tight bilaterally. This describes the athletic muscle-bound body, with symmetrical tightening of the quadriceps, hamstrings, and buttock muscles, which cause the loosening of L4/5 disc joints. When the hips are muscle bound, keep the focus on the balance of your clock face, while performing your stretches to protect your back. Begin with the Basic Low Back Sequence on page 23 and the Hip Sequence on page 56, and spend an excessive amount of time performing the lunges, both kneeling and standing. Then proceed through all of the sequences in this book.

Type 4. One side SI ligaments and muscles are tight—the opposite side SI ligaments and muscles are loose. This type occurs after a fall or an accident that jams one side, such as falling on and breaking the tailbone; repetitive actions involving one side that becomes tight, including habitual leg crossing; or it may be caused by an underlying joint pathology. This is the most common type of SI joint disturbance where the tightness of one side produces the compensatory looseness of the other. The individual might be very athletic or not, and present a leg length discrepancy, one short leg and one long leg. The loose side is usually the painful side, although the pain can travel side to side.

Type 4 SI disturbance affects 30 percent of the population. For yoga practitioners, this misalignment tends to surface after a year or two of performing a regular yoga practice. When one leg is short, all the leg muscles surrounding the leg and pelvic floor on that side will be short and involved to varying degrees. Extreme stretching, or stretching without proper alignment, perpetuates the muscular imbalances until the SI joints register discomfort.

All the muscles of the hip joint are affected, including the psoas and low back muscles. If the right side is jammed, the quadriceps and related muscles on that side would become excessively tight and fixed, while the muscles of the other side, or looser side, would become longer and weaker. Hence, the pain arises on the looser side, as those muscles are straining to maintain stability. The problem is on the right, even though the pain may be felt on the left.

Oftentimes, a Type 4 SI joint disturbance can be coupled with spastic piriformis syndrome. Anatomists have also documented that in 30 percent of the population, the sciatic nerve passes through the middle of the piriformis muscle, rather than passing over it. This may explain how a spastic piriformis muscle can impinge on the sciatic nerve, creating what is called false sciatica. A large portion of the poses that follow will explore how to address a Type 4 SI joint disturbance.

Five Muscle Tests

One of the challenges to finding proper muscular and pelvic balance is to find an objective measure to clarify for our minds the best way to proceed. The following five tests will help you measure and identify which muscles of the pelvic ring are shorter to help guide you when doing your poses. The tests are best done with the help of a friend or family member. Make a note of the measure of each test at the start of your practice so you are able to re-test at a later time and compare. Use the Test Sheet for Muscular Balance on page 138 in Part 4.

Note: Even though the tests look like yoga poses, they are not to be done as yoga poses. Simply get into the position and measure each one.

1. Chair Test: Chair Pose (Utkatasana Variation)

Measures the tone and stability of your pelvic ring and pelvic floor, and the ability for you to transfer your weight without external aide.

Stand with your feet 2 inches in front of the chair and 6 inches apart. Hold your elbows level to the floor. With your spine as straight as possible and your feet flat on the floor, sit down. A straight spine shows functional stability in the pelvic ring. Measure the degree of forward bend in the spine when you sit, or note a sudden collapse into the chair toward the end of the sit. Any angle less than vertical indicates weakness and instability of the pelvic ring and floor, as well as does any rocking that's required when you stand back up.

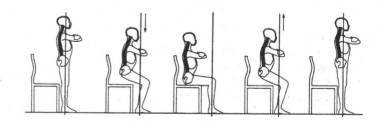

Note angle of spine off vertical

Score: _____

2. Hamstring Test: Head to Knee Pose (Janu Sirsasana)

Measures the ability to flex at the hips, which indicates hamstring length.

Sit on the floor with one leg out straight and the sole of the opposite foot touching the inner knee. Keeping the hips square, reach forward toward your toes. Keep your neck and head in line with your spine. *Do not* round over. Stop at the first sign of restriction. Measure the height of the head to the knee. Compare sides.

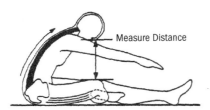

Left leg out: _____

Right leg out: _____

3. Gluteus Test: Supine Twist (Supta Marichyasana III)

Measures the ability to adduct the leg, which indicates the tone of the gluteal muscles.

Lie down on your back; bend one knee and place the toes under the straight knee. With your opposite hand holding your mid-thigh, draw the knee slowly across your body until you feel limited by a feeling of tightness or discomfort. Keep your shoulders down. Compare the tightness of each side by noting how far across the mid-line the knee passes. Note: Avoid rolling onto the right hip as shown in the image.

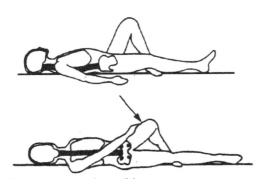

Distance across the mid-line

Left hip: _____

Right hip: _____

4. Quadricep Thigh Test: Half Frog (Ardha Bhekasana)

Measures the ability of the leg to extend, which indicates the length of the quadricep and illio-psoas muscles.

Lie down on your belly. Keeping the pelvis grounded by pressing the pubis into the floor, grab one ankle behind your back and draw the heel toward the same buttock. Measure the distance from the foot to the buttock and compare sides to discover the tighter side.

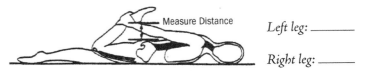

Left leg: _____

Right leg: _____

5. Groin Test: Bound Angle Pose (Baddha Konasana)

Measures the ability of the leg to abduct and shows the openness or lack of openness of the inner leg.

Sit with your back straight against a wall on one or two blankets, bring the soles of the feet together, heels close to your groin, and let the legs fall out. Measure and compare the distance of the knees from the floor. If keeping your spine straight while drawing your heels close in is difficult while you're on the floor, then sit in a chair, bring the soles of your feet together on the chair seat, and measure the height of the knees to the floor. In some cases, you may need to have a second chair in front of you to hold your feet.

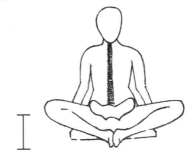

Measure height of knees

Left knee: _____

Right knee: _____

4 Practice Guidelines Toward a Balanced Pelvic Ring

Here are four steps to help you make friends with your hips, pelvic floor, and sacroiliac joints, and build your awareness.

Step 1: Demonstrate to yourself the discrepancies between the two sides by administering the *five muscle tests*.

Step 2: Help yourself "feel" the imbalances with the Hip Sequence on page 56.

Step 3: Learn to focus your practice to unwind the short side, as well as tone and stabilize the long side. The poses on the shorter side typically will be held a bit longer, or the pose may need to be repeated a second time on that side alone to create length. The opposite applies when a long muscle needs to be shortened and toned. You would repeat the poses that tone those muscles, rather than stretch them. One key is to create pelvic floor symmetry left and right.

Step 4: Use the pose Stand Tall, or Tadasana, as home base. Start with your feet hip-width apart and knees bent to level the pelvis front to back and left to right, i.e., balance your clock face. Place your hands on your hips for reference; the focus is to keep the hips level as you straighten the legs. Observe the ease or difficulty in doing so as you return to this pose throughout your yoga practice.

Balancing Sacroiliac Joint Asymmetry

The first step always to relieve back pain is to create length and space, followed by creating relative muscular balance, and then by building muscle tone. The four pose lists that follow are grouped based on those principles, in that order. The first sequence provides length and space while creating some muscle tone that will stabilize a wobbly sacrum. The second sequence, called the Sacral Un-sticking Sequence, addresses the muscular imbalances in our pelvis that often result in pinching and discomfort in the SI joints, hips, low back, groin, or knees. The third, Balancing the Pelvic Floor Sequence, is designed specifically for those students who suffer from a Type 4 sacroiliac imbalance, and will help create balance. The fourth set of poses offers progressions for toning the pelvic floor and pelvic ring. These pose sequences have been chosen because they offer the most direct action on the pelvic ring, which includes all the muscles of the hips, thighs, and low back. They'll help you identify reliable ways to practice and move yourself toward pain relief, find pelvic floor balance, create pelvic tone, and discover sacroiliac joint stability.

There are times when it's necessary to employ the assistance of other professionals, such as physiatrists, chiropractors, physical therapists, cranial-sacral therapists, or knowledgeable yoga teachers to help us on our healing journey. Remember to practice mindfully, avoid a pose if it causes more pain, and ask for assistance.

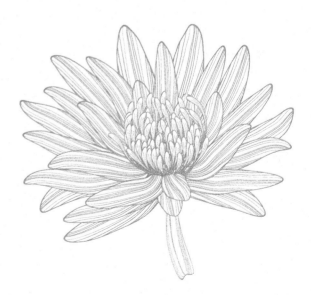

Sacral Stabilization Sequence

This particular sequence is ideal for persons who have Type 1 sacroiliac instability. When the sacroiliac joints (SI joints) are irritated, I recommend you practice only the vertical, front to back poses, which are listed in this sequence, with no twists or lateral poses of any kind. Practicing this sequence is estimated to take 30–40 minutes after you're familiar with the poses. When practice time is at a premium, adjust by ending your practice after pose 7. And as always if one or two of the poses give you good relief, feel free to practice those regularly.

POSE 1. **STAND TALL / TADASANA**

Presented here is a variation of the pose practiced with a block between the feet. The block will act as reference in order to help you find the lift of your pelvic floor, and therefore the lift of the inner body.

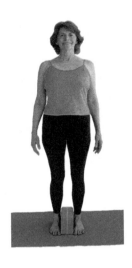

➤**1.** Stand with a block between your feet so both the big toe mound and inner heel make contact. ➤**2.** To lift the inner arches of the feet, bring the inner knee joints forward to face each other, while turning your outer top shins back. ➤**3.** Now squeeze the block with your big toe mounds to move the inner groins back to the center of the pelvic floor. ➤**4.** Reach your heels into the floor as you lift the bottom of your belly up. ➤**5.** Lift your inner body up from your inner leg to your pelvic floor, and from the pelvic floor up to your chest. ➤**6.** Roll your shoulders back and down as you lift the center of your chest high. ➤**7.** Now hug the block with your inner heels to wrap the outer shins and thighs back.

Hint: Be certain to take your top thighs back far enough for your pelvic floor to be in line with the crown of your head. Extend up through your crown.

POSE 2. **FORWARD FOLD / UTTANASANA**

The variation of this pose with the blocks between the feet and the top inner thighs provides insurance that the pelvic floor will be evenly spread, allowing the SI joints the space necessary to find ease.

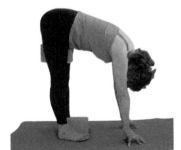

➤**1.** Place a block between your feet and your upper inner thighs. ➤**2.** Hinge forward at your top thighs and place your hands on the floor or on other blocks. ➤**3.** Relax your spine and the back your head and neck. ➤**4.** Micro-bend your knees to avoid hyper-extending, and shift your weight forward so your hips are over your heels. ➤**5.** As you exhale, attempt to lift the block with your inner thigh muscles and move it backwards any amount. Soften your belly forward. ➤**6.** Breathe deeply and relax you arms and shoulders. ➤**7.** Hold for 5 breaths.

Hint: When you shift your hips forward, raise your toes in order to keep sinking your heels into the earth and open the back of your knees without hyper-extending them.

CAUTION: If you feel discomfort in your lower back, raise your chest by placing your hands higher onto the seat or back of a chair. The idea is to make your spine long and flat to avoid pinching that tube.

POSE 3. **STRADDLE FORWARD FOLD—CONCAVE BACK / PRASARITA PADOTTANASANA**

The next two poses are basically the same as when they were introduced in the Leg Toning Sequence, Poses 14 and 15, on page 100. In this pose, bring the clock face parallel to the floor. Maintain a flat spine with the shoulders at the same level as the hips: this is the optimal position for gravity to help the SI joints release.

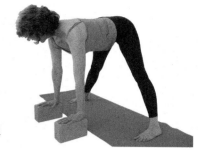

➤**1.** Move into the pose, with your feet slightly pigeon-toed. ➤**2.** Place your hands on your hips to bring your clock face perpendicular to the floor. ➤**3.** Press your heels into the floor and lift your knees and the bottom of your belly strongly up. ➤**4.** As you exhale, hinge at your hips to send your sitting bones back as you extend your chest forward. Keeping your spine extended, place your hands on the blocks. ➤**5.** Inhale and move your breastbone forward and up as you draw your shoulder blades toward your waist, arcing your upper back slightly. ➤**6.** Exhale and lift from the head of the calf to the sits bones to move your top thighs back any amount. ➤**7.** Hold for 3–5 breaths.

Hint: Wrap the skin of your outer shins and outer top thighs back to hold the hips and sacrum stable from side to side.

POSE 4. **STRADDLE FORWARD FOLD—ROUNDED BACK / PRASARITA PADOTTANASANA**

A continuation of the previous pose, this position allows gravity to complete the extension and release of the spine and sacrum, as well as lengthen the hamstring muscles fully.

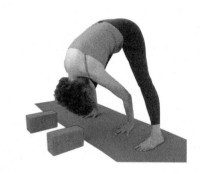

➤**1.** Begin in the flat back position with the hands on the blocks as above. ➤**2.** Exhale and fold forward, hinging at the top thighs, and walk your hands back, keeping your front spine long. ➤**3.** Release your head down. ➤**4.** Shift your weight forward until you feel your heels become light, and then lift your toes to unlock your knees and allow your calves and hamstrings to stretch. ➤**5.** Open from the outer back knees up to your sitz bones, and then anchor the outside edge of your foot. ➤**6.** Draw the outer shins and outer top thighs back to elongate your lower belly forward and down. ➤**7.** Hold for 3–5 breaths. Come out of the pose the same way you went in.

Hint: Feel for the balance of the weight on each foot. Compress your outer shins and outer top thighs in to compact and stabilize your hips from the sides.

POSE 5. **DOWNWARD FACING DOG / ADHO MUKHA SVANASANA**

To help stabilize the sacrum, it's important to learn to use both the inner and outer leg in downward facing dog pose. We know the pose extends the spine by lengthening the arms and the back of the legs; with the help of the block for reference, you'll be able to more fully engage the legs and stabilize your hips. For detailed reminders, please refer to Pose 6 in the Basic Neck and Shoulder Sequence, page 30.

Version B–Hands on the floor

➤**1.** Move into the pose with your feet at the wall and a block between your feet, holding with your inner ankle and heel. ➤**2.** As usual, press your hands down to lift your hips into the air. ➤**3.** Move your pubic bone back between your legs to lift your hips further up, rolling the skin of the buttocks over the sits bones and into the lower back. ➤**4.** Deepen the crease at the top of your thigh and extend up your inner arms. ➤**5.** Keep your heels in contact with the wall, then bring your inner knee forward and your outer knee back. Hug the block with your heels. ➤**6.** Now attempt to wrap your outer top thighs back as much as possible. ➤**7.** Relax your neck and work your legs. ➤**8.** Hold the pose for 5–7 breaths.

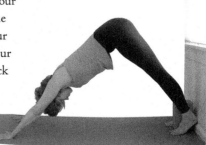

Hint: Reach the little finger forward as you draw your outer top thighs back. Make the outer back knee and the inner back knee the same distance from the wall.

CAUTION: Those with very short hamstrings will need to keep their knees bent to allow the sitting bones to lift and the sacrum to become part of the spine. Spinal extension is the priority.

POSE 6. **LOCUST POSE / SALABHASANA**

This pose activates all the muscles that hold the sacrum in place, toning the gluteal muscles and hamstrings, and stabilizing your hips. Refer to Pose 10 in Progressive Spinal Extensions on page 82 for more details.

Version B–Legs only

➤**1.** Move into position on the blanket with a belt around your mid calf. ➤**2.** With your hands beside your chest and your toes curled under, lift the inner legs up off the floor, pressing your tail deep in. Draw your shoulder blades and buttocks toward your feet. ➤**3.** With an exhale, lift your toes 2–4 inches off the floor, keeping the legs straight. ➤**4.** Press out on the belt as if to break it; that action will activate and tone the buttock muscles as you lift your inner thighs. ➤**5.** Hold for 3–5 breaths.

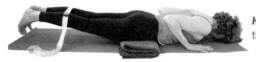

Hint: Open the back of your knee fully by extending in two directions—toward your feet and pulling from the knee up toward your buttocks—to further tone the base of the buttocks and stabilize the sacrum.

POSE 7. **WIDE LEG CHILD POSE / BALASANA**

Release the inner thigh muscles while maintaining a neutral spine so that the sacrum settles toward the floor, returning to its neutral position. For more information, see Pose 11 in Progressive Spinal Extensions on page 83.

➤**1.** With your knees very wide apart, move your hips forward toward your knees to find a neutral spine. ➤**2.** Slowly move your hips back and forth to relax your hips and low back; then find a place to hold the pose keeping your low back flat. ➤**3.** Hold for 5–7 breaths. ➤**4.** Exit the pose slowly, bringing your knees together; then lift your chest.

CAUTION: If your inner thighs are tight, keep your hips forward above your knees. It's more important to keep your lower back neutral in this application than to move your hips toward your feet.

POSE 8. **PELVIC LIFT / SETU BANDHA SARVANGASANA**

In order to fully activate and stabilize your hips and sacrum, this version of the pose using a belt is your best choice. For more Hints and Cautions, please refer to Pose 10 in the Alternate Low Back Sequence on page 40.

Version B

➤**1.** Place a strap around your thighs, 4–6 inches above your knees, and slide your hips toward your feet so your knees are over your ankles. ➤**2.** Curl your tail and slide your knees forward to lift your hips up. ➤**3.** Exhale and press down into your heels to lift the hips higher. ➤**4.** Turn the upper arms under your chest, with the shoulders blades moving toward the spine. ➤**5.** Press your arms down to raise your breastbone toward your chin in order to elongate your spine and protect your lower back. ➤**6.** Repeat the lift 3 times, holding for 3–5 breaths.

Hint: This pose is an excellent choice for persons who experience low back weakness or sacroiliac instability. Be sure to press out into the belt to activate the deep gluteal muscles.

Note: optionally, place a block between your feet to keep them apart.

POSE 9. **YOGA LEG LIFTS / URDHVA PRASARITA PADASANA**

There are three possible methods for doing this pose, all of which are described in Pose 5, Progressive Abdominal Toning, page 35. For this Sequence, I have chosen Version C because it creates optimal length in the spine. The strong lift of the lower belly also stabilizes the front of the sacrum. Remember to build your abdominal tone progressively. If you're not yet ready for Version C then go back to Version A and substitute that version here, as the low back is the most secure in that version.

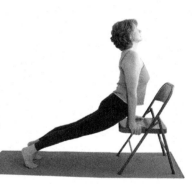

Version C

➤**1.** Lie on your back with your arms extended overhead. ➤**2.** Bend your knees to your chest and extend both legs up. ➤**3.** Keep your head on the floor and extend from your side waist toward your fingers. ➤**4.** Press the back of your palms into the floor to release tension in the neck. ➤**5.** Exhale and lower the legs down as you strongly draw in and up through the center of your clock face. ➤**6.** Repeat for 3–6 rounds.

Hint: When you create full stability of your clock face, your gluteal muscles will also contract.

CAUTION: When you feel your neck tense, know that the center of your clock face has lifted. You'll need to develop more awareness and control of the transverse abdominus.

POSE 10. **UPWARD FACING DOG / URDHVA MUKHA SVANASANA**

Extend the front spine from the pelvic floor to the top chest and tone the back of the body with this dynamic pose. These actions make our spine stronger, and improve posture and organ function. Version B, presented here, gives optimal extension to the spine, and, because the sacrum is part of the spine, gives the best opportunity to decompress and align the sacrum. For more details, see Pose 8 in Progressive Spinal Extensions on page 81.

Version B

➤**1.** Place your hands just in front of your hips on the chair seat, fingers pointing out. ➤**2.** Allow your knees to bend briefly to lift the bottom of your belly in and up toward your chest. ➤**3.** Roll your top shoulders back and press forward with the bottom tips of your shoulder blades. ➤**4.** Then lift your inner thighs up and extend back into your heels as you draw your tail forward and up toward your chest. ➤**5.** Hold the pose for 3–5 even and deep breaths. ➤**6.** Rest and repeat.

Hint: Roll your chest open from front to back by bending your elbows—pretend you're doing the door chest hang—and then straighten your arms and continue with the pose.

POSE 11. HALF SHOULDER STAND AT THE WALL / ARDHA SARVANGASANA

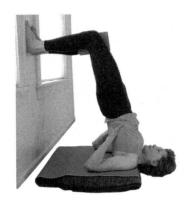

Inverted poses are integral to yoga, and they offer many benefits. Refer to Pose 5 in Six Basic Restorative Poses on page 49. The variation offered here is only one step away from full shoulder stand. Because the feet are on the wall, the weight of the body will stay primarily on the elbows and upper arms, and off the neck. Also, holding a block between the knees will keep the sacrum from wobbling and perhaps pinching. Similar to Upward Facing Dog Pose, you'll experience optimal extension in the spine. In this pose, gravity is helping to traction the sacrum, making it more likely to reseat itself into alignment.

Choose cotton or wool blankets that are firm and stack easily without slipping. Fold them so they're wider than your shoulders, stacking three or four with the folded edges together, to create a height of 3–4 inches. If, when you lie flat with your head off the blanket, your buttocks are also off the blankets, consider placing blocks under your hips to keep your spine neutral.

➤**1.** Place the stack of folded blankets approximately 1 foot away from a wall, with the folded edges together and facing away from the wall. ➤**2.** Lie down on the blankets with your buttocks close to the wall and your head off the blankets and on the floor. Place your neck half on and half off the edge of the blanket. ➤**3.** With your knees bent and your feet on the wall, place a block between your knees. ➤**4.** With an exhale, lift your hips up the same as you would for a pelvic lift, lifting from the tailbone. ➤**5.** Interlace your fingers and stretch your arms behind you. ➤**6.** Press your forearms down to turn the upper arms out and under so you stand on your shoulders. ➤**7.** Lift your shoulder blades and your chest. ➤**8.** Bend your elbows and place your hands as high up your back toward your shoulders as possible, with your fingers pointing up. ➤**9.** Lift the head of your tail strongly up as if to lift the sacrum up out of your shoulders. ➤**10.** Soften the sides of your neck and let your chin lift and be light. ➤**11.** Hold the pose for 2–4 minutes. ➤**12.** To come out, release the hands, roll down, and then slide back away from the wall until your shoulders and spine are off the blankets. ➤**13.** Bring the soles of your feet together at the same height as your hips, and relax in Supine Bound Angle Pose.

Hint: Do your best to stand on the top edge of your shoulders, as that will take the pressure out of the neck and head. To support the lift of your chest, squeeze your elbows in toward each other, and then pin the shoulder blades to your back ribs.

POSE 12. SUPINE BOUND ANGLE POSE / SUPTA BADDHA KONASANA

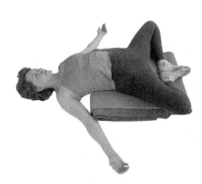

This pose is similar to the Supine Bound Angle found in the Sacral Un-sticking Sequence on page 118. The difference here is that the pelvis and feet are elevated on the props, level with each other, and higher than the shoulders. The connection of the feet allows the thighbones to relax in their sockets, while the muscles of the inner legs have the opportunity to let go evenly. This horizontal spreading of the belly will help to relax the SI joints and quiet the stimulation resulting from the previous pose.

➤**1.** Slide into the pose after half shoulder stand, as described above. ➤**2.** Hold the position for 2–3 minutes, and then lie flat with your legs extended in Corpse Pose for 2 minutes.

Sacral Un-sticking Sequence

These simple poses will serve as first aid when your sacro-iliac joints feel "out of sorts" and should provide relief. This is an excellent practice choice for those with Types 2, 3, and 4 SI joint disturbance. Practice the poses in the order presented for optimal results. Remember to give more time to your tighter areas. The one pose you can do any time, anywhere for quick relief is Pose 8, the "Sink Stretch." The whole sequence is estimated to take 30–35 minutes once you're familiar with the poses.

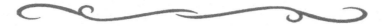

POSE 1. **TRACTION STRAP STRETCH I, II, III / SUPTA PADANGUSTHASANA**

Please refer to Pose 1 in Progressive Spinal Extensions on page 75 for directions on how to place the lower belt, as well as hints and cautions. Then proceed to practice Strap Stretch I and II, and then progress to the variation offered here for the third position.

Strap Stretch III—variation

➤**1.** Begin with both legs fully extended, reaching into the belts. ➤**2.** Keep your clock face balanced so the outer hip of the upper leg is moving away from your waist. ➤**3.** Yield to the traction on your spine by allowing your top thigh to be pulled away from your belly as you draw the bottom of the belly in and up. ➤**4.** When you begin to take the leg across the midline, keep your hips solidly on the ground. ➤**5.** Hold for 3–5 breaths and repeat.

Hint: If you go too far into the pose, your knee may want to bend. Do your best to maintain the extension of the whole limb and progress slowly. If the stretch is particularly painful on one side, rhythmically move in and out of the stretch using your breath before holding the pose.

Inner Action: Spread the sole of your foot and reach out to extend both the inner and outer line of the leg.

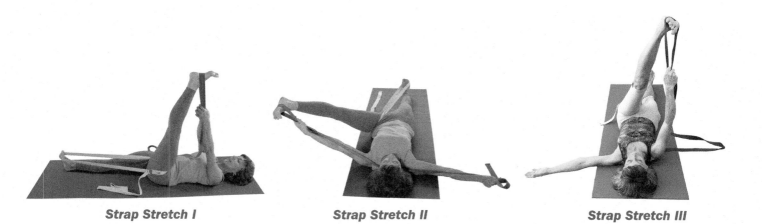

Strap Stretch I **Strap Stretch II** **Strap Stretch III**

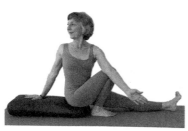

POSE 2. **SEATED CLOSED TWIST / MARICHYASANA III**

Perform Version B of the closed twist, with the arm to the outside of the knee. Please refer to Pose 4 in the Shoulder Toning Sequence on page 85 for directions. To adapt this pose for pelvic floor balance, we'll modify it by narrowing the pelvic floor when twisting toward the long leg side and widen the pelvic floor when twisting toward the short leg side.

Version B–Adapted

➤**1.** Begin sitting on a bolster or two blankets with your legs out straight. ➤**2.** Bend the short leg and place the foot with the toes even with the opposite knee. ➤**3.** Use your hand to broaden the pelvic floor sideways *only when the short leg is bent.* ➤**4.** Lift your spine and lengthen the sides of the body. ➤**5.** Turn your belly toward your knee to cross your arm to the outside. ➤**6.** Maintaining the lift of your spine, press the arm into the knee and knee into the arm to twist. ➤**7.** When you *twist toward the long leg side*, contain the pelvic floor by tucking the hip in toward the midline. ➤**8.** Hold each side for 3–5 breaths. ➤**9.** Repeat the twist on the tighter or short leg side a second time.

POSE 3. **SEATED TRACTION TWIST / MATSYANGASANA**

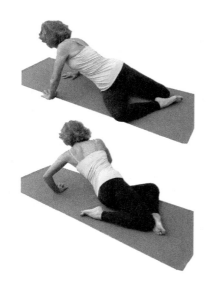

In this pose the small muscles along the spine are released, the psoas muscle is lengthened and released, the length of the spine is maintained, and the spine is encouraged to go back into alignment with itself.

➤**1.** Sitting on the floor, fold your right leg and place the foot next to your hip, with the toes pointing straight back. ➤**2.** Place the arch of the left foot in contact with your right kneecap, like a cup and saucer. ➤**3.** Resting the left thigh on the floor, walk your hands around behind you to the left and away from your pelvis. Allow your right hip to lift. ➤**4.** Lift your left hip and slide the flesh of your buttocks straight toward your left ankle. ➤**5.** Extend your right knee into the floor as you lift from the bottom of your belly to your chest to lengthen the front spine. ➤**6.** As you exhale, twist your spine like a spiral from the bottom to the top. ➤**7.** Hold for 3–5 breaths.

Hint: It's helpful to bend the elbows slightly to lengthen and turn the spine simultaneously. Be mindful to lengthen both sides of the spine evenly, especially the side closest to the floor.

CAUTION: To avoid any pain in the knee, be certain to fold the knee evenly, aligning the heel with the center of the buttocks, before swinging the foot alongside the hip.

POSE 4. **HIP STRETCH FLEXED /ARDHA AGNISTAMBASANA**

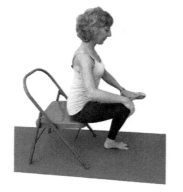

Poses 4 and 5 here are variations of the classic pose and are so important to practice because they develop our ability to externally rotate the thigh in the hip joint in both flexion and extension. These are the first movements a person looses when the hip joints are degenerating. Practicing these poses will go deep into the small muscle attachments around the hip joint, creating more opening and mobility. Be certain that you do complete the Hip Sequence on page 56 at least once a week. Be mindful—application is everything.

Version B

➤**1.** Sit toward the front of the chair with your spine straight. ➤**2.** Place your right ankle on your left knee with your foot flexed. ➤**3.** Sharpen your sitz bones as you work to turn the outer knee toward the floor. ➤**4.** Breathe deeply into your hips and hold for 30–60 seconds. ➤**5.** Repeat each side twice.

Hint: It's important to keep the ankle of the right foot square to prevent any over stretching and instability in the knee joint.

POSE 5. **HIP STRETCH EXTENDED / UTTHITA AGNISTAMBASANA**

Version B

➤**1.** Sit toward the front of the chair with your spine straight. ➤**2.** Place your right ankle on your left knee with your foot flexed. ➤**3.** Lean back in the chair so you feel you're slumping. ➤**4.** Place your left hand on your belly, and with your right hand, grasp the inner right thigh at the knee. ➤**5.** As you exhale, simultaneously turn the right thigh out and down as you lift your lower belly in and up, using your hands. ➤**6.** Hold for 3–5 breaths. Change sides.

Hint: Feel free to move the left foot more under the chair seat to give gravity more of a chance to draw the right leg down.

Note: When sitting in the chair, you can combine poses 4 and 5 above. Progress your pelvis in three positions: a) Draw your navel in and tip your pelvis back to release the upper thigh out toward the knee and down. b) Sit upright. c) Bend slightly forward into flexion.

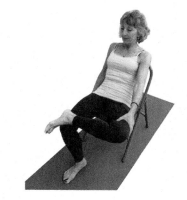

POSE 6. **SINK STRETCH**

I call this pose "first aid" for the sacroiliac joints because it can be easily done in any location with or without our yoga clothes on! The value in both versions of this pose is the way they extend the spine and open the hips, allowing the sacrum to often reseat itself into a place of ease. The sacroiliac joints sit to the front or inside of the pelvic bones. Therefore, by extending the spine and making our clock face parallel to the floor, gravity will aid the release of the sacrum, allowing the spine and the use of our hips to pull the sacrum into better position.

Version A

➤**1.** Begin with your feet slightly wider than your hips. ➤**2.** Bend your knees to a half squat or enough so you feel the weight of your buttocks. ➤**3.** Hold onto a sink, doorknobs or other secure prop. ➤**4.** Step your feet back until you feel the full extension of your spine, arms fully extended, back flat. ➤**5.** Now sharpen your sitz bones and reach them back as if they were being pulled. ➤**6.** Hold for 3–5 breaths.

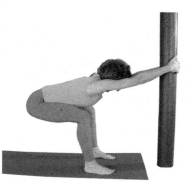

Hint: Using your breath, traction your spine back to allow the root of your thighs to be heavy; then roll the skin over your buttocks toward your lower back.

Version B

➤**1.** Come to a flat back half squat without holding onto anything. ➤**2.** Place your hands to the sides of your knees and create isometric resistance by pressing in with your hands and out with your knees in order to spread and widen your top thighs—in essence, opening the pelvic floor. ➤**3.** Roll the flesh over your buttocks to make the sitting bones sharp. Also, extend your front spine to maintain a flat back. ➤**4.** Sink the midpoint of your sacrum toward the floor to gap the joints and provide relief. ➤**5.** Hold for 3–5 breaths. Repeat as necessary.

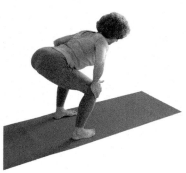

Hint: Your hands are pressing in on your knees and your knees are pressing out; however the knees don't move—only the top thighs spread apart.

POSE 7. **PELVIC LIFT / SETU BANDHA**

Practice Version B of this pose, with a yoga belt placed 4–6 inches above the knees, with the knees hip-width apart. Refer to Pose 8 in the Sacral Stabilization Sequence, page 112, or Pose 10 in the Alternate Low back Sequence, page 40, for more detailed instructions.

➤**1.** Move your body into the pose as shown in the photo. ➤**2.** Press your arms down to raise your breastbone toward your chin in order to elongate your spine and protect your lower back. ➤**3.** Then press out on the belt to awaken and tone the buttock muscles of the weaker side. ➤**4.** Hold for 3–5 breaths and repeat.

Hint: Give particular attention to activate the buttock muscles on the weaker side. Think of pressing your heels down to pull up from the back of your knee to your buttocks, and also pull the buttocks toward the back of your knee.

POSE 8. **SUPINE BOUND ANGLE / SUPTA BADDHA KONASANA**

As there are many ways to practice a yoga pose, here's a simple version of reclined bound angle pose that adds traction using your hands and breath. The traction will be felt along the psoas and the sacral ligaments that are located deep in toward the back of the abdomen. Refer to Pose 8 in the Sacral Stabilization Sequence on page 00 for other information.

➤**1.** Lie flat on the floor with the soles of your feet pressed together and your knees wide. ➤**2.** Use your hands on your top thighs and press them away from your side waist as you draw the bottom of your belly in and up. ➤**3.** As you inhale, pause; as you exhale, press your thighs and lift your belly to traction your sacrum and spine up into the chest region. ➤**4.** Repeat 4–6 times.

Hint: Your hip bones stay flat and steady on the floor. The only lifting is of the internal organs and muscles of the lower belly.

Balancing the Pelvic Floor Sequence

The pelvic floor is not an area of the body that we typically give much attention to, unless there is a problem. We know that the pelvic floor holds our organs in place, houses the poop shoot and urinary track, and correlates to the health of our sexual organs. We know that we can create tone by practicing Kegels and avoid incontinence, yet rarely do we consider that the pelvic floor could be out of balance. The main muscle of the pelvic floor is the perineum. In a Type 4 sacroiliac disturbance, the perineum will be shorter and tighter on one side. The pose sequence that follows will help you open the short side of the perineum, giving more mobility to the hip and sacrum on that side, and creating more space and ease, so the other muscles of that side can begin to release as well.

Observe how in this sequence I ask you to return to Stand Tall, Tadasana, several times to evaluate the movement toward a balanced pelvis, reflecting Step 4 of your Practice Guidelines Toward a Balanced Pelvic Ring outlined on page 109.

Sometimes when we perform a pose, the pelvic ring may go more out of balance, yet another pose may put the pelvis back in balance. Observe which poses put you out of balance. Check yourself on your clock face positioning and your alignment, and use patience in creating muscle length in those poses. Depending on how deep your imbalance is, you might choose to practice this sequence two or three times a week, interspersing with other foundational sequences like the Hip Sequence on page 56, Progressive Spinal Extensions on page 75, Leg Toning Sequence on page 94, and others.

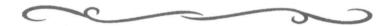

POSE 1. **STAND TALL / TADASANA**

To establish the position of the pelvis, start with your feet hip-width apart and your knees bent to level the pelvis front to back and left to right—in other words, balance your clock face. The focus is on keeping the hips level as you straighten the legs. See Pose 1 in the Sacral Stabilization Sequence on page 110.

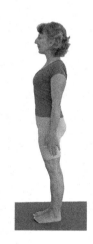

➤**1.** With a block between your feet and knees bent, place your hands on your hips for reference.
➤**2.** Squeeze the block with your big toe mound to move the inner groin back to the center of the pelvic floor. ➤**3.** Reach your heels into the floor as you lift the bottom of your belly up to flatten your clock face. ➤**4.** Slowly straighten your knees and make your pelvis stay level as best you can. Then wrap the outer shins and thighs back to also hug the block lightly with your heels. ➤**5.** Now lift your inner body up from your inner legs to your pelvic floor, and from the pelvic floor up to your chest.

Hint: Feel how activating the outer leg creates stability in the hips.

Note: Block between feet not shown in photo.

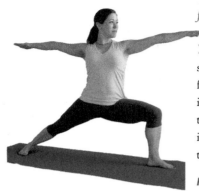

POSE 2. **SIDEWAYS LUNGE / VIRABHADRASANA II**

The lateral standing poses help to open the hips and the pelvic floor particularly on the straight leg side. For a full description, refer to Pose 7 in the Leg Toning Sequence on page 96.

➤**1.** After turning your feet, work the inner groin of the rear leg back until you feel your buttocks blossom to the back. ➤**2.** Keeping the inner groin back, lift the bottom of your belly and draw the buttock flesh back down to point your tail toward the floor. ➤**3.** Keep the hips level to the floor by *strongly* lifting the pubis and inner groin of the front leg until that sits bone is directly under the hip as you bend that knee. ➤**4.** Extend from the left inner groin toward your knee and turn the skin of the knee from inside out. ➤**5.** Maintain the back leg and pelvis as you coil your left (front) hip into its socket and lift that inner groin up. ➤**6.** Reach into your back leg and arm and hold for 5–7 breaths.

Hint: Press the rear thigh out away from the midline to broaden the pelvic floor when the straight leg is the shorter leg.

CAUTION: DO NOT square your hips to the side of your mat. Attempting to square your hips is likely to create distress in your hip, sacral, and knee joints. Allow the right hip to move slightly forward so it points in the same direction as the toes of that foot.

Note: Practice this pose with the rear heel against a baseboard/wall. Use the wall for resistance to press the inner rear thigh toward the outer rear thigh and open the pelvic floor on that side.

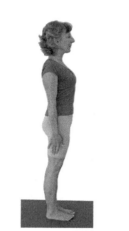

POSE 3. **STAND TALL / TADASANA**

Repeat the bent knee entry from Pose 1 to re-establish the position of the pelvis and balance your clock face. Compare the clock face of each Tadasana to the one before to track the balance and re-balance of the pelvis.

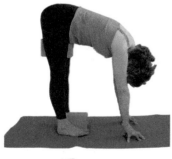

POSE 4. **FORWARD FOLD / UTTANASANA**

The variation of this pose with the block between the top inner thighs ensures that the pelvic floor will be evenly spread, allowing the SI joints the space necessary to find ease.

➤**1.** Place a block between your feet and your upper inner thighs. ➤**2.** Hinge forward at your top thighs and place your hands on the floor or on blocks. ➤**3.** Relax your spine and the back of your head and neck. ➤**4.** Micro-bend your knees to avoid hyper-extending and shift your weight forward so your hips are over your heels. ➤**5.** As you exhale, attempt to lift the block with your inner thigh muscles and move it backwards any amount. Soften our belly forward. ➤**6.** Hug the block between your feet with the big toe mounds as you begin to fully straighten the legs. ➤**7.** Breathe deeply and relax your arms and shoulders. ➤**8.** Hold for 5 breaths.

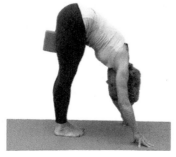

Hint: When there is a leg length discrepancy, the inner thighs will have different levels of muscle tone. Watch to see which inner thigh moves back first by noticing the angle of the block. Do your best to move the block back evenly, taking both inner groins to the center of the thigh as when you Stand Tall / Tadasana.

CAUTION: Mind your back. If you feel any negative or questionable pain in your lower back while in this pose, please raise your hands up higher onto your shins or a chair. Protect your back by lengthening your spine toward a flat back.

Note: Please remove the block between the feet if you can pull your feet closer together, which makes the top block more effective. As shown in the second photo.

POSE 5. SIDEWAYS LUNGE WITH A CHAIR / VIRABHADRASANA II

The variation of this pose with the bent leg foot on a chair helps to both spread the pelvic floor on the short side as well as coil and shorten the pelvic floor on the long side. For a full description, refer to Pose 7 in the Leg Toning Sequence on page 96.

Short Leg Side

➤**1.** Place the back of the chair against a wall for safety and stand one leg length away with your side to the chair. ➤**2.** Place the foot of the short leg on the seat with your heel hooked on the edge. ➤**3.** Repeat the actions of the pose, lifting the lower belly, drawing the mid buttocks down, and turning the ribs to face forward. ➤**4.** Turning the skin of the knee from the inside out, bend the knee until it's above your ankle. ➤**5.** Keeping the rear leg thigh pressed back, squeeze in on the mid-buttock of the bent leg and strongly lift your lower belly. ➤**6.** Hold for 3–5 breaths, rooting down into your straight leg heel and lifting your spine.

Hint: Be certain to bend the front knee to be above the anklebone or slightly forward to release and soften the short side of the pelvic floor when that leg is on the chair.

Long Leg Side (shown in the photo)

➤**1.** Place a strap loop around the top of the thigh with the buckle on the outside so that the long end goes under the thigh and can be held against the opposite hip. ➤**2.** Follow the same steps 1–5 as you did with the short leg foot on the chair. ➤**3.** Holding the strap in the hand of the straight leg, use the opposite hand to help guide the bent knee to turn from the inside out. ➤**4.** Exhale and use the strap to pull the top of the thigh down and under as you spread across the front pelvis to the opposite hip. This will help pull the long loose hip into its socket. ➤**5.** Again, exhale and activate the straight leg. Press the inner thigh out to anchor the outside edge of the foot. Feel the spread of the pelvic floor on that side. ➤**6.** Sustain the pelvic actions for 3–5 breaths.

Hint: As the legs work together, the more you lift the corner of the pubis on the long leg side, the more the short leg side will pull toward the center. Therefore, maintain the actions of the long bent leg pulling into the hip socket, and also focus on pressing the inside of the straight leg (i.e., the short side) wide as you root down into that outer heel.

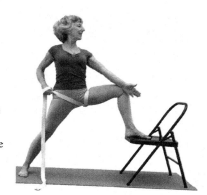

POSE 6. SIDE ANGLE POSE WITH A CHAIR / PARSVAKONASANA

The actions of the hips and thighs are the same as in the previous pose in regards to the short side–long side. The benefit of this pose is in how it extends the side ribs and waist while toning and balancing the legs.

Long Leg Side

➤**1.** Follow steps 1–5 in the previous pose. ➤**2.** Exhale and reach your left arm out to extend your left side, and then place your hand on the chair in front of your shin. ➤**3.** Swing your right arm forward and up alongside your ear. ➤**4.** As you exhale, press your arm into your knee to coil your left hip deep into the hip socket. ➤**5.** Lift the bottom of your belly toward your chest, and then turn your chest to face forward. ➤**6.** On your next exhale, root down into the outside of your right foot and lift the palm of your hand up out of your hip. ➤**7.** Hold for 3–5 breaths.

Short Leg Side

➤**1.** Follow steps 1–6 as you did on the long leg side. ➤**2.** Hold for 3–5 breaths.

Hint: Be aware of the differences of the two sides and work toward balance.

Inner Action: In other words, bring the hip of the bent long leg side as deep in and under as you can, while pressing the short leg side away from the mid-line. When the short leg is bent, release the top thigh downward and lift your belly while firming the thigh and gluteal muscles of long straight leg.

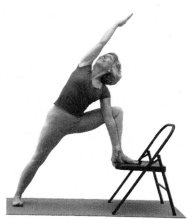

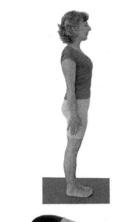

POSE 7. **STAND TALL / TADASANA**

Repeat the bent knee entry from Pose 1 to re-establish the position of the pelvis and balance your clock face. Press the big toe mound into the block to move your inner groins back, and then wrap the outer shins and thighs back to also hug the block with your heels. Lift the pelvic floor strongly up. Check the changes in hip level.

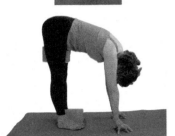

POSE 8. **FORWARD FOLD / UTTANASANA**

Repeat Pose 4 from this sequence. The variation of this pose with the block between the top inner thighs ensures that the pelvic floor will be evenly spread, allowing the SI joints the space necessary to find ease.

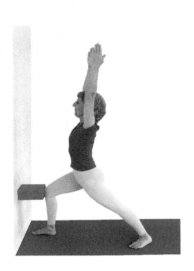

POSE 9. **STANDING LUNGE / VIRABHADRASANA I**

Remember, the most stable version of the Standing Lunge for the SI joint is Version B, where you face a wall with a block in front of the bent knee. Hold the pose longer when the shorter or tighter leg is the straight rear leg. See Pose 5, Progressive Spinal Extensions, page 79, for more details.

Version B

➤**1.** Place a foam block at the wall so you can hold it in place with your right kneecap, positioning your ankle below your knee. ➤**2.** Take a large step back with your left leg and place that foot so the heel is slightly turned in. ➤**3.** Turn your hips to face forward, squaring the clock face toward the wall. ➤**4.** Press your knee into the block as you lift the right side of your pubis strongly up to balance 3:00 and 9:00. ➤**5.** Root down through the outer rear heel as you press that outer hip in toward the midline. ➤**6.** Raise your arms and spine up and extend your arms out of your hips. ➤**7.** Hold for 3–5 breaths and change sides.

Hint: Strongly lift the bottom of your belly in and up toward your chest to lift both corners of your pubic bone and flatten your clock face. This action will stabilize and lift the spine from the front of your SI joints as well as support your lumbar spine.

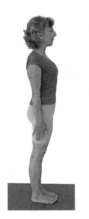

POSE 10. **STAND TALL / TADASANA**

Repeat the bent knee entry from Pose 1 to re-establish the position of the pelvis and balance your clock face. Press the big toe mound into the block to move your inner groins back, and then wrap the outer shins and thighs back to also hug the block with your heels. Lift the pelvic floor strongly up. Check for balance.

POSE 11. **STRADDLE FORWARD FOLD—CONCAVE BACK / PRASARITA PADOTTANASANA**

Again, this pose will help to activate the legs evenly and spread the pelvic floor, release the hips, allow the sacrum to settle toward the floor, and create length in the spine. For more details, refer to Poses 14 and 15 in the Leg Toning Sequence on page 100.

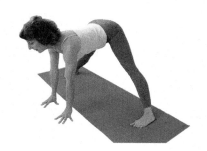

➤**1.** Position your feet evenly, with the toes turned in. ➤**2.** After lifting up through your legs, hinge slowly forward from the hips. As if the block were between your thighs, move your inner groins and thighs back evenly to keep the clock face even. ➤**3.** Soften your belly and evenly extend both sides of your waist forward, with the top thighs pressing back. ➤**4.** Continue extending your front spine as much as possible. ➤**5.** Hold for 3–5 breaths.

Hint: Feel for the balance of the weight on each foot. If you are heavy on the outside of one foot and the inside of the other foot, chances are your hips, clock face, and sacrum are not level. Try to turn the top thigh in on the side with the lighter inner foot. Use a hand behind you to feel for the levelness of your hips so your clock face remains parallel to the floor.

POSE 12. **STRADDLE FORWARD FOLD—ROUNDED BACK / PRASARITA PADOTTANASANA**

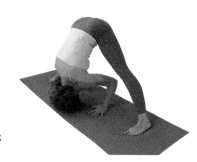

➤**1.** From the concave back above, exhale and release your spine down without shifting your weight back. ➤**2.** Place your hands even with or slightly in front of your feet. ➤**3.** Lift your shoulders up as your hands root down. ➤**4.** Now lift from the back knee up and over the top buttocks. ➤**5.** Keep your belly soft and breathe. ➤**6.** Hold for 3–5 breaths.

CAUTION: As always, if rounding forward causes any pinching along your spine or hip areas, remain in the concave back position, Pose 11..

Hint: Place your hands on your outer shins. Then press in on the mid-shin with your mid-palm as you broaden the backs of your top thighs evenly. This brings even width to the pelvic floor, allowing the spine and sacrum to release further.

POSE 13. **CHAIR POSE / UTKANASANA**

Although this pose looks like we are about to sit in a chair, the real translation is "fierce pose," because it generates strength and heat. Practice this to build the tone of both sides of the pelvic floor, the lower abdominals, and balance the clock face. The pose is added here to act as a stabilizing and counterbalancing pose in this sequence. It will be repeated again in the next section.

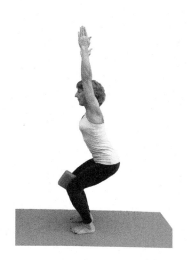

➤**1.** Stand Tall, and then place a block in its narrow position between your knees. ➤**2.** Place your hands on your hips, and flatten and lift the center of your clock face. ➤**3.** Bend your knees as if to sit deep in a chair. ➤**4.** Draw your knees back so you can see your big toes, tilting your body forward to a 45-degree angle. ➤**5.** Squeeze the block with your inner knees to lift your inner groins and the bottom of your belly in and up. ➤**6.** Wrap the flesh of your outer thighs around and under you to make an invisible chair. ➤**7.** When you're steady, raise your arms overhead and extend your spine. ➤**8.** Maintaining the squeeze of the block, hold the pose for 3–5 breaths.

Hint: With a leg-length / pelvic-ring discrepancy, one side of the pubis may be more difficult to lift as well as to wrap the outer thigh under you. Focus your attention on that looser side, using the squeeze of the block to access those muscles.

CAUTION: Do not allow the inner groins to drop lower than the outer groins, as this will place too much pressure in the lower back.

Progressive Pelvic Ring Toning

After creating length and space along with relative muscular balance, we're ready to begin building the necessary muscle tone to stabilize and make our hips more fully functional. There are several poses offered here; however, no one is expected to perform all of these poses at one time. I often give the first two poses—Chair Pose and Tree Pose—as homework to my classes because they're efficient at maintaining the tone of the pelvic floor and lower abdomen.

Select one or two poses to practice for a week, and then rotate poses from week to week. Again, you may find certain poses in the list that are more helpful to you than others—certainly practice those more often. Hold each pose to your capacity. Listen to your body, be your own best friend. When you start to quiver or shake, the muscles are showing signs of fatigue. Better to hold for several short rounds than overexert for one long round. If you find your hips or back in negative pain the next day after doing these poses, go back to creating length and space with the Sacral Un-sticking Sequence on page 115 in this section.

After practicing some of the poses listed here, try repeating the Chair Test on page 107, to see what improvement may be coming. Feel free to intersperse any of these poses into your other yoga routines, knowing that they'll give you the tone you need to feel stable and pain free.

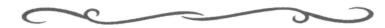

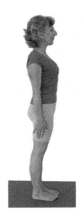

POSE 1. **STAND TALL / TADASANA**

Begin with bent knees to establish the position of the pelvis, and then straighten the legs fully.

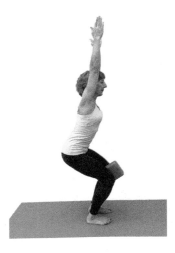

POSE 2. **CHAIR POSE / UTKATASANA**

Build the tone of both sides of the pelvic floor and clock face. Follow the instructions from Pose 12 in Balancing the Pelvic Floor in the previous section, page 123.

➤**1.** Place the block between your knees and hands on your hips. ➤**2.** Draw your knees back and sit deep.
➤**3.** As you wrap the outer thighs under you, scoop your lower belly in and up. ➤**4.** Hold for 3-5 breaths.

Hint: With a leg-length / pelvic-ring discrepancy, one side of the pubis may be more difficult to lift as well as to wrap the outer thigh under you. Focus your attention on the looser side, using the squeeze of the block to access those muscles.

CAUTION: Do not allow the inner groins to drop lower than the outer groins, as this will place too much pressure in the lower back.

POSE 3. **TREE POSE / VRKSASANA**

This simple pose can help reinforce and train the muscles of the inner and outer leg, as well as the pelvic floor to become stronger.

➤**1.** Begin with your feet together and Stand Tall. ➤**2.** Lift the bottom of your belly and press your mid-buttocks deep in. ➤**3.** Lift the inner legs from the inner ankle up though the pelvic floor to the chest. ➤**4.** Keep the full length of the left inner leg as you transfer your weight onto that leg. ➤**5.** Squeeze in with your outer left hip to stabilize the leg as you place your right foot on the inner thigh. ➤**6.** Micro-bend the standing leg to keep from hyper extending the knee and again strongly lift the inner leg and lower belly up through the pelvic floor to your chest. ➤**7.** Hold for 3–5 breaths and change legs.

Hint: If balance is a challenge for you, raise your right foot up off the floor any amount to place it on your calf, knee, or thigh.

Note: To develop your balance, stand arms-distance from a wall. Lift the leg closer to the wall and place it on your thigh, and then squeeze in with the outer thigh of the standing leg. As you progress, slowly lift your fingers off the wall.

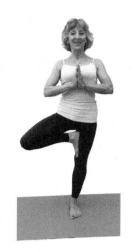

POSE 4. **LOCUST POSE—LEGS ONLY / SALABHASANA**

One way to address a Type 4 sacral imbalance is to practice Locust Pose in an unbalanced way to create balance. This approach will help tone the piriformis and buttock muscles on the long leg side, allowing the short leg side to begin to let go and come to balance. See Pose 10 in Progressive Spinal Extensions, page 82, for more details.

Version G–One leg lifts, then both

➤**1.** Lie down on your belly with your hips on a folded blanket and your chin or forehead on the floor. ➤**2.** Place your hands beside your chest or under the front of your hips and curl your toes under. ➤**3.** Lift the inner thighs up off the floor, and then press your tail deep in. ➤**4.** Draw your shoulder blades and buttocks toward your feet, keeping the inner legs lifted. ➤**5.** On an exhale, lift your long leg 2–4 inches off the floor and stretch your leg back, while pulling the hamstring up into the buttocks. ➤**6.** Hold for 3 breaths. Repeat 2–3 times to tone the loose side. ➤**7.** One time, lift both legs together 2 inches off the floor.

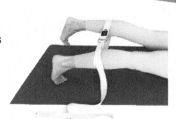

Hint: Be certain to open the backs of the knees in two directions so the base of the buttocks activates to hold the legs just a few inches off the floor.

CAUTION: If you feel any negative pain or pinching in your low back, raise your hips up onto a bolster so you can press your tail down enough to lessen the curve of your lower back.

Version G–Variation with a belt

Using a belt can help connect the thighs to improve the tone of the posterior pelvic ring.

Note: When the calves are belted, loosen the belt so the legs are somewhat wider than hip width. Lift the looser leg higher and press out on the belt to activate both sides of the pelvic floor.

POSE 5. **LOCUST POSE—CHEST ONLY / SALABHASANA**

Remember that the SI joints sit to the front or inside of the pelvic bones. In order to affect an adjustment to the sacrum and create stability and release, it's helpful to use resistance and leverage like we did in the "Sink Stretch" in the Sacral Un-Sticking Sequence, Pose 6, on page 117. It takes effort to elongate your spine and draw the sacrum along with it. Using a belt creates resistance and stability of the base so you can more easily draw your belly and sacrum forward as part of the spine.

This variation of Version A is particularly helpful for people who have a Type 1 or 2 sacroiliac dysfunction. For more details on this pose, see Pose 14-D in the Shoulder Toning Sequence, page 90, or Pose 10-A in Progressive Spinal Extensions, page 81.

Version A–Using a belt

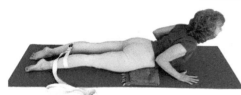

➤**1.** Perform the pose with the front hips elevated on a folded blanket or bolster to get optimal abdominal length. ➤**2.** Strap your shins so they are hip-width apart, and press out strongly in order to move your sacrum deep in. ➤**3.** Keep your feet on the ground and curl your chest up. ➤**4.** Draw your hands back to pull your chest, belly, and sacrum forward. ➤**5.** Work the pose for 3–5 breaths, rest then repeat.

Hint: Make the effort to pull your chest and sacrum forward as you press out against the belt to fully activate your gluteal and sacral stabilizing muscles. Inhale wait—exhale extend.

POSE 6. **UPWARD FACING DOG / URDHVA MUKHA SVANASANA**

From Locust Pose, you can move easily into Upward Facing Dog as a continuation, or practice the poses separately, taking a short rest in between. Whether you choose to practice Version A or B of this pose, be certain to put your hands on blocks or higher, until you can easily activate your gluteal muscles. For full details, refer to Pose 8 in Progressive Spinal Extensions, page 81.

Version A–Legs on bolster, hands on blocks

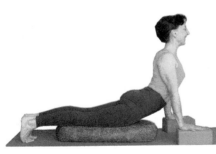

➤**1.** Move into the pose. ➤**2.** Curl your toes under, firm your thighs by straightening your knees, and press your tail down into the bolster. ➤**3.** Inhale and roll your shoulders back and draw your breastbone forward. ➤**4.** Continue to reach back through your heels and ground down through your tailbone as you straighten your arms as much as possible, lifting your chest. ➤**5.** Hold briefly and repeat 3–5 times.

Version B–Hands on a chair

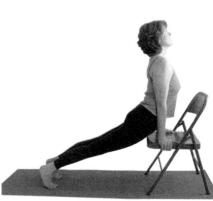

➤**1.** Move into the pose, allowing your knees to bend briefly to lift the bottom of your belly in and up toward your chest. ➤**2.** Roll your top shoulders back and press forward with the bottom tips of your shoulder blades. ➤**3.** Reach your legs back and lift your inner thighs up any amount. ➤**4.** Extend back into your heels as you draw your sacrum in and up toward your chest. ➤**5.** Breathe and hold the pose for 3–5 breaths. Then rest and repeat.

Hint: Curl the whole spine as best you can. Lengthen your front spine from the bottom of the belly to the bottom tip of the breastbone and then curl the upper chest back.

Inner Action: Take your sacrum deep in and lift your spine up through your chest as you extend the legs back.

POSE 7. **DOWNWARD FACING DOG / ADHO MUKHA SVANASANA**

When you choose to practice several of the toning poses presented above, your body will require some form of counterbalancing pose to relieve the gluteal and back muscles after their work and return the muscles to neutral. As these poses are likely to leave you with some post-exercise discomfort the next day, it's important to return the muscles to neutral to minimize or remove that discomfort. I am suggesting Downward Facing Dog pose first as it's the complement to Upward Facing Dog. You might also substitute Wide Leg Child's pose, or Supine Bound Angle Rock, as your counter pose.

➤**1.** From a kneeling position, press up, moving your pubic bone back between your legs to lift your hips up into the pose. ➤**2.** Wrap your outer armpit toward the floor and lift the inner arm to release strain in the shoulders. ➤**3.** Reach the fingers forward as you press the top thighs back to continue extending your spine. ➤**4.** Hold for 5–7 breaths. Repeat 3 times.

Hint: To more deeply release your lower back, reach your heels back and down closer to the floor.

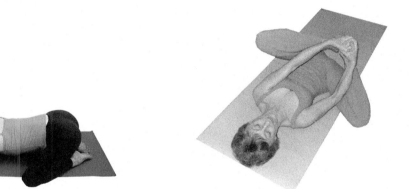

Wide Leg Child's Pose   **Supine Bound Angle Rock**

part 4

Bonus Section

Take advantage of two additional concise sequences to improve posture and rejuvenate after hours at the computer! You will also find a table of poses to help you customize your personal yoga practice.

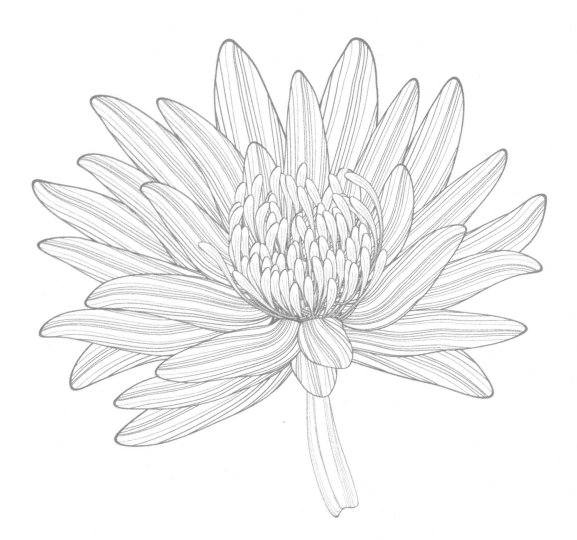

Computer Recess: A Floor Sequence

As a yoga teacher and healing guide, I have been amazed at the amount of hours required to sit at a desk to write this book. This has given me a new appreciation for the dilemma of many of my students who are required by their jobs to sit for up to 8 hours a day. Because our bodies really thrive on movement, sitting for long hours is problematic for our hips, backs, shoulders, and arms. This sequence was created to counterbalance the muscular imbalances of sitting in a chair.

Whether you work in an office or at home, you can continue to learn about your body and be your own best friend by taking time to practice these poses. I have indicated how each pose in the sequence will help you return your body to balance. This sequence can be done in the morning before sitting, at lunchtime, or in the evening after a day of sitting for simple and fast relief. Expect to complete the sequence in 15–20 minutes, ideal for a short recess!

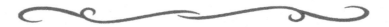

POSE 1. TRACTION TWIST / SUPTA MATSYANGASANA

The anatomical action here is internal rotation of the thigh. This pose stretches the front of the thigh, and both the long and the short psoas muscle, as well as offers traction for the lumbar spine. See Pose 1 in the Basic Low Back Sequence on page 23 for more guidance.

➤**1.** When you drop your knees to the left, keep your right knee in line with your nose. Your pelvis will lift up about halfway. ➤**2.** Extend the top thigh away from your hip as you curl your tail toward your pubis and draw the bottom of the belly in and up. ➤**3.** Hold for 3–5 breaths on each side, and repeat.

Hint: Protect the knee by drawing the toes toward the shin. A 90-degree angle of thigh to shin is the ideal.

Inner Action: As you reach the inner knee out and down toward the floor, scoop your lower belly in and up, and then turn your belly away from the knees.

POSE 2. PELVIC LIFT / SETU BANDHA SARVANGASANA

To encourage optimal length and release in the psoas muscles, please modify the pose in this way: lift your hips only halfway up to allow the psoas muscles to hang like a hammock holding your internal organs. This pose extends the front thigh and psoas muscles, and tones the buttock muscles. See Alternate Low Back Sequence page 40 for more details.

➤**1.** With the block in place, move into the pose. ➤**2.** Curl your tail and slide your knees forward to lift your hips halfway up. ➤**3.** Turn the upper arms under your chest, shoulders blades moving toward the spine. ➤**4.** As you lift the hips up firm the buttocks and keep the lower belly concave and soft. ➤**5.** Hold the lift for 5–7 breaths. Repeat three times.

Hint: Peel the spine up off the floor, extending the knees slightly forward. Roll down slowly, with the back of the waist touching before the hips. Moving in this way will encourage the release, integration, and balance of the psoas muscles.

Note: If you are able to raise your buttocks high up, then press your arms down to raise your breastbone toward your chin in order to elongate your spine and protect your lower back.

POSE 3. **BASIC LYING TWIST / JATHARA PARIVARTANASANA**

After a long time sitting at a desk, you can tone the internal/external obliques and loosen the spine and shoulders with the basic twist. For more details, see Pose 1 in the Basic Neck and Shoulders Sequence, page 28.

Version A

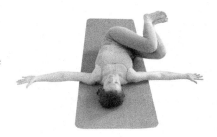

➤**1.** Extend your arms fully, with the knees toward your chest higher than your navel. ➤**2.** As you exhale and twist, keep the knees 6–10 inches off the floor. ➤**3.** Again exhale, drop the lower belly in, and turn your bottom ribs from the center of your clock face to the left. ➤**4.** Use your exhale to move you in and out of the pose. ➤**5.** Hold for 1–2 breaths and repeat 3–5 times.

CAUTION: If your low back is very stiff or unstable, carry your knees half way to the side or less. Stop when your opposite ribs begin to lift from the floor.

Version B

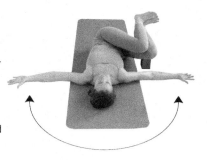

➤**1.** Place the knees down onto blankets or a block to prepare for arm circles. ➤**2.** Reach out with your left arm and describe a half circle past your right hip to your right hand. ➤**3.** Keep your neck relaxed and extend your left arm from the shoulder until both palms touch. ➤**4.** Continue sweeping the arm over your head along the floor to finish the second half of the circle back to the starting position. ➤**5.** Repeat, making 3 full circles in one direction and then in the opposite direction. ➤**6.** Pull your knees in toward your chest and back to center. Change sides.

CAUTION: If your shoulders are particularly tight, you may not be able to touch the floor above your head. In that case, simply rotate the outer arm and shoulder toward your face, extend out, and allow your arm to float above the floor. Find the place of stability and ease.

POSE 4. **YOGI CURL-UPS**

Curl-Ups tone the abdominal muscles, including the rectus abdominus, transverse abdominus, internal and external obliques, as well as the psoas muscles. Poses 4 and 5 use reciprocal inhibition to release the muscles in the back of the neck and chest. Refer to Pose 1 in Progressive Abdominal Toning, Versions A and C, on page 33 for more guidance.

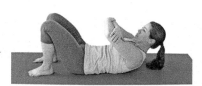

➤**1.** Hold your elbows in front of your chest, OR cross your arms behind your head, as needed to support your neck. ➤**2.** Curl up one third of the way, eyes gazing at your knees. ➤**3.** Hold for 3–5 breaths. Repeat 2–3 times. ➤**4.** For Version C, add a twist by bringing the left shoulder toward your right knee, and then your right shoulder toward the left knee. ➤**5.** Hold each side 3–5 breaths. Repeat 2–3 times.

Hint: Keep the center of the pelvic clock on the floor and your inner groins soft.

Note: In Version A, hold your elbows and curl up so the bottom back ribs are on the floor and the shoulders are off.

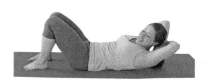

Hint: Keep the center of the pelvic clock on the floor. In the twist observe which side seems weaker, and hold that position longer.

Inner Action: As you exhale and twist, connect the bottom front ribs to the opposite inner groin.

Note: In Version C, when you twist, one shoulder blade will touch the floor and the other will be off the floor.

POSE 5. **SUPINE HEAD LIFTS**

This pose is a great neck toner, countering the effects of working at a computer. Practice the pose by lifting first to the center, and then to the left and right. See Pose 3 in Basic Neck and Shoulder Sequence, page 29, for more information.

➤**1.** Move into position on the mat. ➤**2.** Exhale and lift your head to gaze at your toes, keeping your shoulders relaxed. ➤**3.** Hold for 10 counts, and then rest. ➤**4.** Repeat 3 times. ➤**5.** Now repeat the pose, turning your head right for 5 counts, returning to center, and then to the left for 5 counts.

CAUTION: When turning your head, always deliberately return to the center before lowering your head to avoid unnecessary strain. If your neck feels weak, opt to do one side at a time, resting for 2 breaths in between sides.

POSE 6. **HALF FISH POSE / ARDHA MATSYASANA**

This pose tones the back of the neck, the rhomboids, and the mid-trapezium to relieve upper back and neck strain. Refer to Pose 4 in Basic Neck and Shoulders Sequence, page 29, for more details.

➤**1.** Move into the pose, lifting your chin until the back of your crown is in contact with the floor.
➤**2.** Press the back of your head and elbows down to engage the muscles of your upper back and neck to lift your chest up, forming an even arc from the top of the neck to bottom of your shoulder blades.
➤**3.** Pressing the outer edge of the elbow firmly into the floor, broaden your collarbones and draw the inner shoulder blades farther away from your neck. ➤**4.** Hold for 7 breaths. Repeat 3 times.

Hint: Be sensitive to the back of your neck—sometimes less is more. Better to lift your chin only 1 inch and create an even arc of the neck, rather than collapse the tube of your neck by throwing your head back too much and risk pinching nerves.

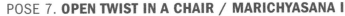

POSE 7. **OPEN TWIST IN A CHAIR / MARICHYASANA I**

This version extends the pectoralis major and minor muscles, releasing all front shoulder and chest muscles, and relieving tension in the neck. See Pose 6 in Progressive Twists, page 65, for more details.

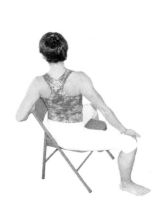

➤**1.** Sit in the chair as shown, legs apart at 90 degrees, chest lifting to move your spine in and up.
➤**2.** Place your left hand inside the left knee, straighten the arm and roll your shoulders back.
➤**3.** Bend your right arm and draw the elbow way back to place the hand against the outside of the chair back. ➤**4.** Turn your chest any amount toward the chair back to leverage your front chest open.
➤**5.** Reach your bent elbow back as you lift and press your chest forward. ➤**6.** Use the leverage of both arms to draw the shoulder blades down and pin them to your back ribs. ➤**7.** Hold for 3–5 breaths and repeat on the other side.

Hint: Extend your bent elbow diagonally away from your back so as to maintain space between the two shoulder blades. Use your breath to help lift and widen your front and back chest.

POSE 8. **REVERSE PLANK / PURVOTTANASANA**

This pose is a weight-bearing pose that opens the front arm and top chest, relieving thumb pain/strain, and toning the back body. See Pose 7, Version A, in Progressive Spinal Extensions, page 80, for more guidance.

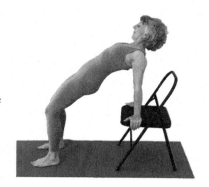

➤**1.** As you push up into the pose, be sure to keep the soles of your feet pressing down. ➤**2.** Inhale as you slide your hips forward and up, lifting your chest. Look straight ahead or release your head back. ➤**3.** Exhale and return your hips to the chair. ➤**4.** Repeat 3 times. ➤**5.** On the 4th time, hold the pose for 3 breaths.

Hint: Extend your fingers sideways to activate the muscles of your back arm and shoulder blades.

Inner Action: Extend down into the heel of your hand to lift your side chest as much as possible to lengthen your front arm.

Remember: Keep your shoulder blades pinned and your top chest lifted, no matter how high your hips lift.

POSE 9. **DOWNWARD FACING DOG / ADHO MUKHA SVANASANA**

Choose Version A or C of this classic pose. Remember, the goal is to extend and lengthen the legs, arms, spine, and chest by extending the back of the legs or hamstrings, the para-spinal muscles, the latissimus and arm muscles, and tone the serratus anterior muscles to stabilize the shoulder joint. See Pose 15 in Alternate Low Back Sequence on page 43 for more details.

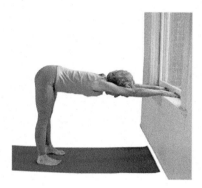

Version A
➤**1.** Stand with your feet hip-width apart. ➤**2.** Hinge forward from the front of your hip joint and reach your arms out to touch a wall or a ledge. ➤**3.** Keep your spine long by moving your breastbone forward and your sits bones back. ➤**4.** Lift your sits bones any amount to stretch the back of your legs. ➤**5.** Wrap your outer armpit toward the floor and lift the inner arm to release strain in the shoulders.

Version C
➤**1.** Place the blocks on the lowest level, hip-width apart against the wall. ➤**2.** Start on your hands and knees, with your feet close to the blocks; then walk your hands 6 inches forward of your shoulders. ➤**3.** Press your hands down to lift your hips into the air. ➤**4.** Place one foot at a time on a block with your toes reaching off the edge and your heels touching the wall, with the foot at a 45-degree angle. ➤**5.** Press the inner palms and index knuckles down to extend up your inner arms to your hips. ➤**6.** Deepen the crease at the top of the thigh, and then roll the skin of the back leg over your buttocks to extend the back of your legs and spine. ➤**7.** Anchoring your heels to the wall, slowly straighten your legs as much as possible. ➤**8.** As your heels press into the wall, lift up from your mid-calf to your buttocks. ➤**8.** Relax your neck. Hold the pose for 5–7 breaths.

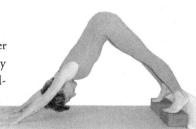

Hint: Those with very short hamstrings will need to keep their knees bent. Spinal extension is the priority.

POSE 10. **LOCUST POSE / SALABHASANA**

All versions of locust pose create tone in the back body, which extends the spine to give us strength to stand tall. See Pose 10, Progressive Spinal Extensions, page 82, for more information.

Version A–Chest only

The preliminary action of lifting only the chest in this variation reverses the forward curl of the spine from long hours of sitting. The pose gradually tones the spinal muscles, mid-trapezius, and rhomboid muscles to lengthen the front body.

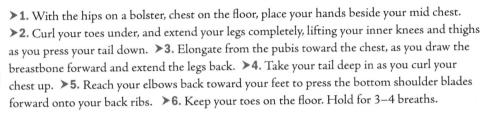

➤**1.** With the hips on a bolster, chest on the floor, place your hands beside your mid chest. ➤**2.** Curl your toes under, and extend your legs completely, lifting your inner knees and thighs as you press your tail down. ➤**3.** Elongate from the pubis toward the chest, as you draw the breastbone forward and extend the legs back. ➤**4.** Take your tail deep in as you curl your chest up. ➤**5.** Reach your elbows back toward your feet to press the bottom shoulder blades forward onto your back ribs. ➤**6.** Keep your toes on the floor. Hold for 3–4 breaths.

Hint: The more you extend back through your legs, the more you'll be able to expand your chest forward. Watch for the less moveable parts of your spine and do your best to curl all parts of the spine equally.

Version B–Legs only

Practicing this pose with the legs only will more heavily weight and tone the hamstrings, buttocks, and low back.

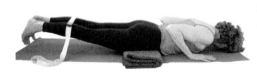

➤**1.** With the belt in place, feet approximately hip-width apart, lie down with your hips on a folded blanket and your chin or forehead on the floor. ➤**2.** Place your hands beside your chest and curl your toes under. ➤**3.** Lift the inner leg up off the floor, and then press your tail deep in. ➤**4.** Draw your shoulder blades and buttocks toward your feet keeping the inner leg lifted. ➤**5.** With an exhale, lift your toes 4–6 inches off the floor, keeping the legs straight. ➤**6.** Press out on the belt as if to break it in order to continue pulling the buttock muscles toward your feet and activating your gluteal muscles and hamstrings. ➤**7.** Hold for 3–5 breaths.

Inner Action: Extend out the heels as you pull up from the back of the knee toward the buttocks, toning the hamstring muscles. Keep the buttocks moving toward your feet.

POSE 11. **WIDE LEG CHILD'S POSE / BALASANA**

A counter-balancing pose to release and relax the spine after locust pose, this will stretch the inner leg, as well as relax the low back and gluteal muscles.

➤**1.** Take your knees very wide apart. ➤**2.** Begin with your hips forward toward your knees to bring your spine to neutral, and then slowly move your hips back and forth until your hips and low back relax. ➤**3.** Find a place to hold the pose without rounding your low back, resting your forehead and elbows on the folded blanket. ➤**4.** Hold for 3–5 breaths. ➤**5.** To come out of the pose, slowly bring your knees together and lift your chest.

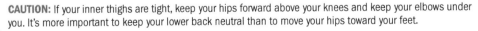

CAUTION: If your inner thighs are tight, keep your hips forward above your knees and keep your elbows under you. It's more important to keep your lower back neutral than to move your hips toward your feet.

Posture Sequence

Posture is a concern for most adults, especially as we get older. As with all of yoga, to reap the benefits, practice is required. If our goal is to have better posture, we need to reinforce muscle memory through repetition. In this section you will find six poses that require only about 15 minutes of your time, yet will leave you with a feeling of being more upright, optimistic, and satisfied.

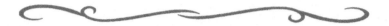

POSE 1. **ALTERNATE KNEES TO CHEST /APANASANA**

Condition your psoas muscle gradually by lifting one leg at a time up and down. This way of practicing uses the weight of the legs to both lengthen and evenly tone the psoas muscles, relieving strain in the lower back.

➤**1.** Lie flat on your back with your legs out straight. ➤**2.** Draw your right knee into your chest, keeping 3:00 and 9:00 level. ➤**3.** Extend out the straight leg and press it down onto the floor. ➤**4.** As you inhale, lift the straight leg up as far as posible without tilting the clock face. ➤**5.** As you exhale, slowly lower the leg 6–10 inches from the floor, paying special attention to pulling the center of your clock face in and up. ➤**6.** Repeat the straight leg lift 3–6 times. ➤**7.** Change sides and repeat.

Hint: Find the sweet spot for the bent leg by turning your knee to point toward your armpit rather than into your chest.

CAUTION 1: If lifting the straight leg causes any back pain, simply begin by bending and drawing the knee in toward the chest before straightening the leg toward the ceiling. Lower the leg on the exhale and repeat.

CAUTION 2: If you aren't able to lower the leg to 6 inches from the floor while keeping the center of the clock face drawn in and up, only go as far as you can, or place your foot on a block and practice lifting your foot an inch off the block by activating the center of your clock face.

POSE 2. **BASIC LYING TWIST / JATHARA PARIVARTANASANA**

The following pose will help to tone the diagonal stomach muscles, and the internal and external obliques.

➤**1.** Lie on your back, stretch your arms out to either side to make a "T" shape, and bend your knees in toward your chest. ➤**2.** Keeping the knees closer to your chest than the navel, roll over your hip to twist your knees to the right any amount, 6–10 inches off the floor. ➤**3.** Press the back of the right arm down and extend out the left to keep your shoulders in contact with the floor. ➤**4.** As you exhale, drop the lower belly in and turn from the center of your clock face to the left. The lower belly turns one way and the upper belly turns the opposite. ➤**5.** Repeat with the knees dropping to the left. ➤**6.** Hold for 3–5 breaths.

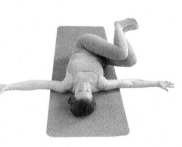

Hint: When you feel sensations along your spine, be confident that reciprocal inhibition is working for you. The sensations are an indication of tension and spasm leaving your back muscles.

CAUTION: In the beginning less is more. Complete the twist with the knees as high as 10-12 inches from the floor. As you progress your body will allow your knees to lower to 6-10 inches off the floor without strain. As always, listen to your body.

POSE 3. **PELVIC LIFTS / SETU BANDHA SARVANGASANA**

Open the front of your hips and thighs with this pose, which lengthens the quadricep muscles, tones the gluteal muscles, and integrates the psoas muscles on both sides. The length of the psoas muscle is a primary contributor to our ability to stand upright.

Version A–Block between knees

➤**1.** Sitting on the floor with knees bent, align your toes with the edge of your mat or an imaginary line. ➤**2.** Slide your hips toward your feet so your knees are right over your ankles. ➤**3.** Lie on your back with the arms by your side. ➤**4.** Place the block between your knees. ➤**5.** Curl your tail and slide your knees forward to lift your hips. ➤**6.** Press your heels down to lift your hips higher. ➤**7.** Turn the upper arms under your chest, shoulders blades moving toward the spine. ➤**8.** Press your arms down to raise your breastbone toward your chin in order to elongate your spine and protect your lower back. ➤**9.** Repeat the lift three times. Holding for 3–5 breaths.

Hint: To keep your neck in good balance, lift your chin slightly before strongly lifting your chest.

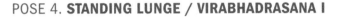

Inner Action: On an exhale, sink your heels and upper arms into the floor and open the back of your knees to further raise your hips and chest.

POSE 4. **STANDING LUNGE / VIRABHADRASANA I**

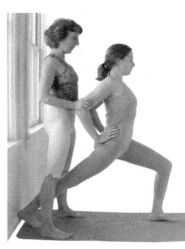

Version C–Heel on the wall

This version of Standing Lunge with the rear heel up on the wall is a good alternative for extending the back leg and spine completely when the calf muscles are short, there has been injury to the knee or ankle, or if the knee or ankle are tender in any way.

➤**1.** Place your left heel up the wall at a 45-degree angle. ➤**2.** Turn you hips to face forward, and step your right foot out as far as possible, keeping your hips square. ➤**3.** Use your hands on your hips to press down as you lift the bottom of your belly in and up to raise your chest. ➤**4.** As you exhale, bend your front knee any amount. ➤**5.** Continue to extend the inner rear heel into the wall as you lift from your pelvic floor to your chest. ➤**6.** Pause on the inhale, extend the leg, and lift your spine with each exhalation. ➤**7.** Hold for 3–5 breaths.

Hint: As you lift the bottom of the belly, the rear knee will want to bend. Maintain the extension of the rear knee and connection of that heel to the wall as you slowly bend the front knee any amount.

POSE 5. **SPLIT LEG FORWARD FOLD / PARSVOTTANASANA**

When you use a wall for this pose, you efficiently lengthen the sides of your spine and the backs of your legs, actions that help you stand taller. The images here show the optimal extension of the spine, as well as the incorrect collapsing of the spine. For best results ask a friend to check your alignment.

➤**1.** Begin in half downward dog pose with your hands on a wall. ➤**2.** Step your right foot forward half way, then step the left foot backward the same amount. ➤**3.** Point the toes of the rear foot out 10 to 15 percent for balance. ➤**4.** Straighten your arms, holding your head even between them. ➤**5.** Press your heels into the floor and draw from the head of your calves toward your hips. ➤**6.** Wrap the outer arms down toward the floor as you lift the inner arms. ➤**7.** Keeping the big toe of the front leg pressing down onto the floor, draw both outer top thighs back to stretch your side waist. ➤**8.** Push your hands into the wall to extend your spine further, drawing your hips back any amount. ➤**9.** Hold for 5–7 breaths. Change sides.

Hint: In order to keep your spine long and straight, please raise your hands higher up the wall until you can practice this pose without rounding and collapsing your back.

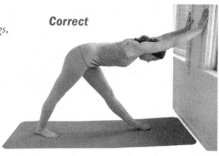

Correct

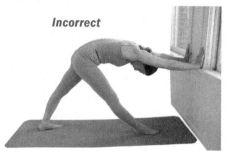

Incorrect

POSE 6. **DOOR CHEST HANG / PURVOTTANASANA**

The door chest hang helps to stretch the large pectoralis muscles of the front chest and lengthen the front of the arms to overcome a rounded chest.

➤**1.** Stand in the center of a doorway. ➤**2.** Hook your fingers around the door jam behind you, placing the base of each palm so it presses out on the inner door. ➤**3.** Bring your armpit chest forward and up as you roll your shoulders back and down. ➤**4.** Lift your navel in and up. ➤**5.** Breathe into the upper chest to stretch the upper front chest and shoulder. ➤**6.** Hold for 60 seconds.

Hint: To increase the stretch, walk your feet forward 3-4 inches, and/or raise your hands up any amount.

CAUTION: If you experience any numbness in your arms, back off 10 percent by lowering your hands, and breathe deeply. Sometimes less is more. Check to see that your top shoulders are rolled back and the bottom tip of the shoulder blades are pinned to your back ribs.

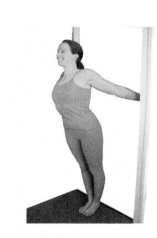

CHOOSING POSES TO CREATE MUSCULAR BALANCE

Listed in order of difficulty from simple to more challenging

MUSCLES / REGIONS	SHORT	LONG
Back Leg / Hamstrings	Strap Stretch I	Pelvic Lifts
	Low Lunge	Locust: Legs Only B
	High Lunge	
	Downward Facing Dog	
	Split Leg Forward Fold	
	Straddle Forward Fold	
	Standing Hand to Foot	
Inner Thigh / Adductors	Strap Stretch II	Lateral Leg Lift
	Kneeling Groin Stretch	Standing Chair Twist
	Bound Angle Pose (sitting)	Standing Leg Stretch w/Twist
	Reclined Bound Angle w/ Support	
	Sideways Lunge	
Front Thigh / Psoas, Quadriceps	Traction Twist	Alternating Knee Curl Ups
	Alternate Knees to Chest w/ Leg Raises	Yogi Leg Lifts – A
	Pelvic Lifts	Chair Pose
	Low Lunge	Boat Pose A, B, C, or D
	Low Lunge: Hands to Knee	
	Standing Scissor Twist at Wall	
	Standing Lunge A, B, or C	
Back / Erector Spinae	Strap Stretch I and III	Open Chair Twist
	Basic Lying Twist	Standing Scissor Twist
	Standing Chair Twist	Locust Pose: Chest Only A
	Closed Twist in a Chair	Upward Facing Dog
	Prone Twist on a Bolster	
Buttocks / Gluteal Group and Piriformis	Basic Lying Twist	Pelvic Lifts
	Strap Stretch I and III	Sideways Lunge
	Hip Stretch Flexed (seated or lying)	Locust Pose: Legs Only

CHOOSING POSES TO CREATE MUSCULAR BALANCE *(continued)*

Listed in order of difficulty from simple to more challenging

MUSCLES / REGIONS	SHORT	LONG
Upper Back and Neck / Rhomboids, Mid Trapezius, Levator Scapulae	Eagle Arms	Closed Twist in a Chair
	Basic Lying Twist w/ Arm Sweep	Half Fish Pose
	Supine Head Lifts	Locust Pose – Chest C, D, E, F
Shoulders–Chest / Pectoralis, Rotator Cuff Muscles	Cow's Head Arms	Closed Twist in a Chair
	Open Chair Twist	Locust Pose – D
	Door Chest Hang	Upward Facing Dog
	Arms Overhead w/ Pole	Sideways Plank
	Elbows on a chair	Seated Closed Twist – B
	Downward Facing Dog	
	Both Arms Extend Back	
	Seated Open Twist B	
	Supported Pelvic Lift	
	Reclined Bound Angle	
Stomach / Transverse Abs, Internal & External Obliques, Rectus Abdominus	Traction Twist	Alternating Knee Curl Ups
	Standing Scissor Twist at Wall	Yogi Curl Ups A, B, C
	Pelvic Lifts	Alternating Knee Curl Ups
	Supported Pelvic Lifts	Basic Lying Twist
	Upward Facing Dog A	Yoga Leg Lifts A, B, or C
Side Body / Quadratus Lumborum, Latissimus Dorsi	Basic Lying Twist	Lateral Leg Lift
	Sideways Chair Twist	Sideways Plank A, B, or C
	Strap Stretch III	Upward Facing Dog A or B
	Side Stretch (standing)	Reverse Plank A
	Downward Facing Dog	
	Standing Leg Stretch w/ Twist	
	Side Angle Pose	
Shoulders & Chest	Cow's Head (Arms)	
	Elbows on a Chair	
	Downward Facing Dog	

Quick Reference Pose Sheets

Here you will find all the sequences offered in this book as simple pose sheets. Once you have learned the particular alignment and actions of each pose, use these pose sheets for quick reference when you practice. Feel free to photocopy these sheets to take with you when you go on a trip. Remember, the benefits of yoga accumulate over time. Continue your practice and enjoy the journey!

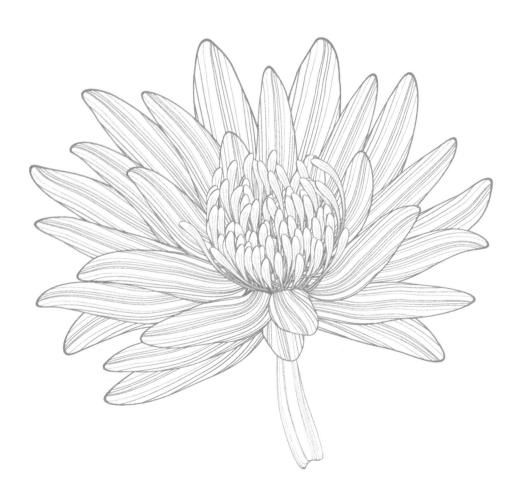

part 5
the short sequences

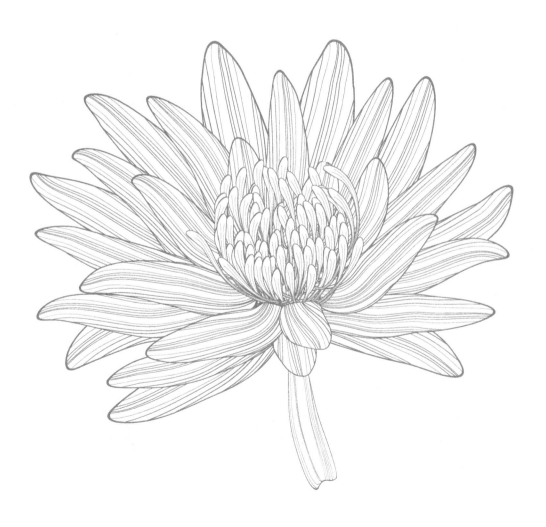

Basic Low Back Sequence Short Form

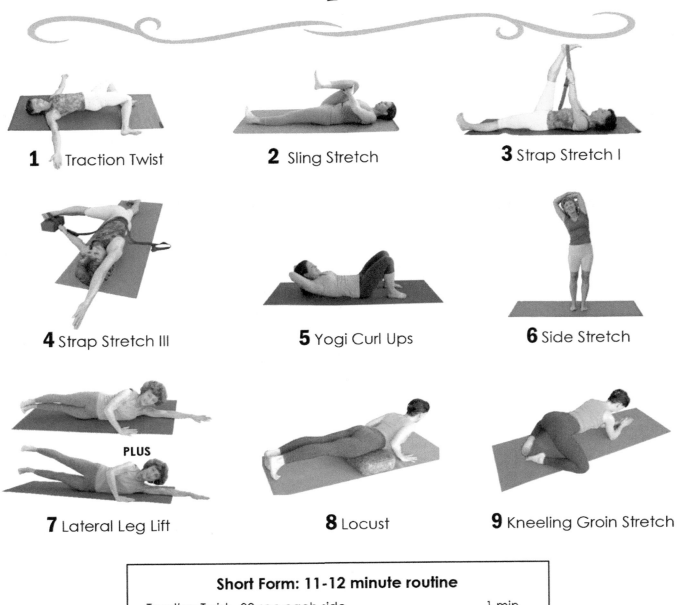

1 Traction Twist

2 Sling Stretch

3 Strap Stretch I

4 Strap Stretch III

5 Yogi Curl Ups

6 Side Stretch

PLUS

7 Lateral Leg Lift

8 Locust

9 Kneeling Groin Stretch

Short Form: 11-12 minute routine

Traction Twist - 30 sec each side	1 min
Sling Stretch - 1 min each leg	2 min
Strap Stretch I - 1 min each leg	2 min
Strap Stretch II - 1 min each leg	2 min
Stomach Strengthener – repeat 3 times	1 min
Side Stretch - 30 sec each side	1 min
Lateral Leg Lift - 30 sec each side	1 min
Locust Pose – repeat 3 times	1 min
Kneeling Groin Stretch - rest for	1 min

Neck & Shoulder Sequence Short Form

1 Sideways Chair Twist   **2** Downward Facing Dog   **3** Eagle Pose (Arms Only)

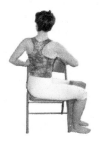

A.

OR

B.

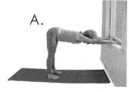

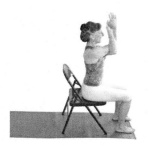

4 Cow's Head - Arms Only   **5** Door Chest Hang

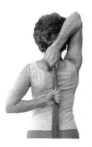

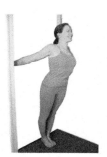

Short Form: 10-12 minute routine	
Sideways Chair Twist – 30 sec each side, repeat	2 min
Downward Facing Dog – 30-60 sec, repeat	2 min
Eagle Pose (arms only) – 60 sec each side	2 min
Cow's Head (arms only) – 60 sec each side	2 min
Doorway Chest Hang – 60 sec	1 min

Hip Sequence

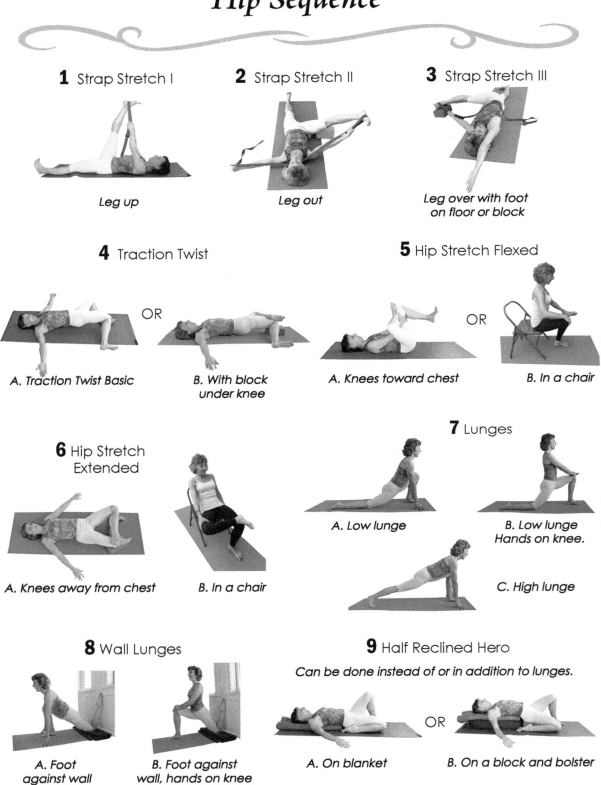

1 Strap Stretch I

Leg up

2 Strap Stretch II

Leg out

3 Strap Stretch III

*Leg over with foot
on floor or block*

4 Traction Twist

OR

A. Traction Twist Basic

*B. With block
under knee*

5 Hip Stretch Flexed

OR

A. Knees toward chest

B. In a chair

6 Hip Stretch
Extended

A. Knees away from chest

B. In a chair

7 Lunges

A. Low lunge

*B. Low lunge
Hands on knee.*

C. High lunge

8 Wall Lunges

*A. Foot
against wall*

*B. Foot against
wall, hands on knee*

9 Half Reclined Hero

Can be done instead of or in addition to lunges.

OR

A. On blanket

B. On a block and bolster

Posture Sequence

1 Alternate Knees to Chest

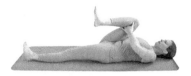

2 Basic Lying Twist

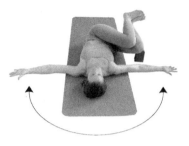

3 Pelvic Lift

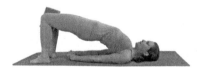

A. Hold block between knees

4 Standing Lunge

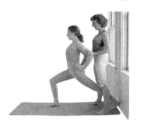

C. Rear heel on wall

5 Split Leg Forward Fold
Hands on wall.

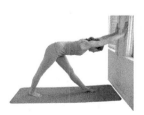
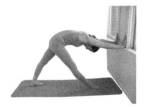

Correct   *Incorrect*

6 Door Chest Hang

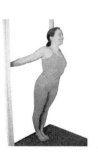

Progressive Pelvic Ring Toning

1 Stand Tall

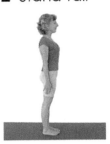

2 Chair Pose

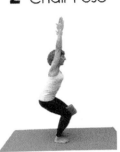

3 Tree Pose

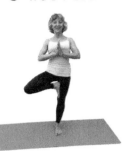

4 Locust Pose Legs Only

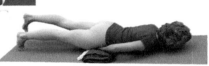

*G. One leg lifts
(with or without belt)*

5 Locust Pose Chest Only

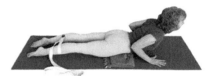

A. Variation with a belt

6 Upward Facing Dog

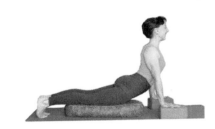

A. Legs on bolster, hands on blocks

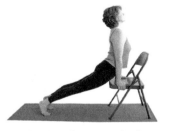

B. Hands on a chair

7 Downward Facing Dog

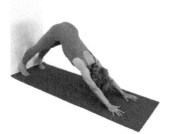

B. Hands and feet down

Sacral Stabilization Sequence

1 Stand Tall

2 Forward Fold

3 Straddle Forward Fold

4 Straddle Foward Fold

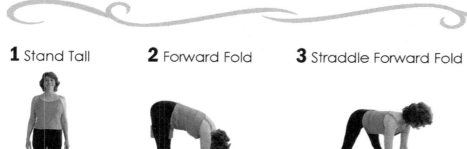

Block between feet

With two blocks

Concave back

Rounded back

5 Downward Facing Dog

6 Locust Pose

7 Wide Leg Child Pose

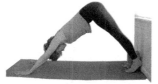
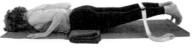
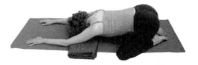

Block between feet

B. Only legs, belt mid calf

8 Pelvic Lift

9 Yoga Leg Lifts

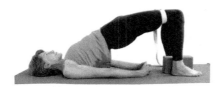
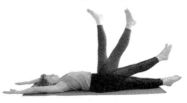

B. Belt above knees, block feet

C. Legs raise and lower, no stops

10 Upward Facing Dog

11 Half Shoulder Stand at Wall

12 Supine Bound Angle

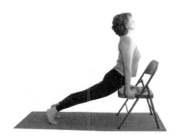
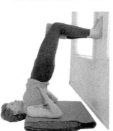
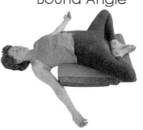

A. Hands on chair

Feet and hips level

the full sequences

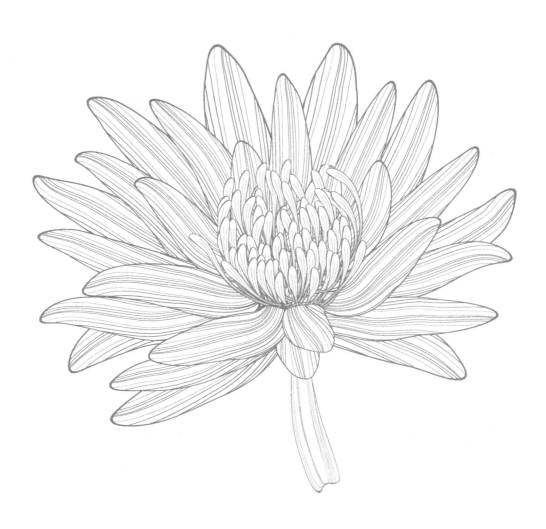

Alternate Low Back Sequence

1 Alternate Knees to Chest

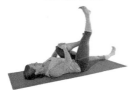

Straight leg up and down.

2 Alternating Knee Curl Ups

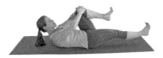

B. One leg extended, long leg up 6-10"

3 Yogi Curl Ups

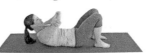

Up in center

AND

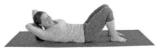

Curl up with twist

4 Basic Lying Twist

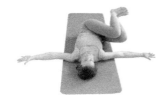

5 Supine Upper Back Twist

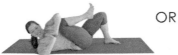 OR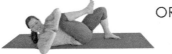

A. Bent knees   *B. Leg extended*

6 Strap Stretch I

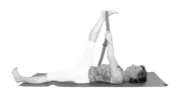

Leg up

7 Strap Stretch II

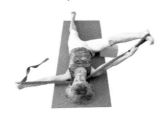

Leg out

8 Strap Stretch III

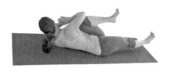

Leg over with foot on floor or block

9 Traction Twist

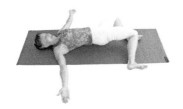

10 Pelvic Lift

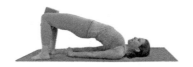 OR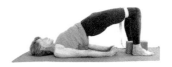

A. Hold block between knees   *B. Belt above knees*

Alternate Low Back Sequence

11 Half Fish Pose

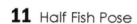

Balance on elbows and back of crown

12 Supine Bound Angle Rock

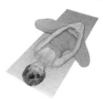

Keep knees wide

13 Downward Facing Dog

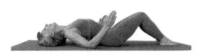

B. Hands and feet down

14 Lunges

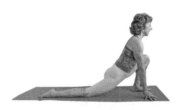

A. Low lunge

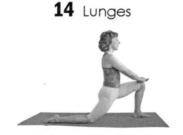

B. Low lunge: hands on knee

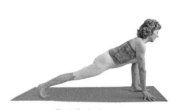

C. High lunge

15 Downward Facing Dog

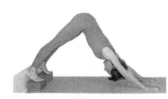

C. Feet on blocks at the wall

OR

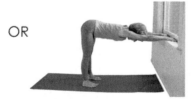

A. Hands on wall

16 Standing Chair Twist

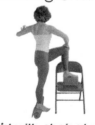

Twist with chair at wall

17 Standing Hand to Foot Pose

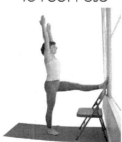

18 Upward Facing Dog

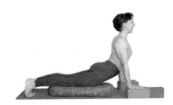

On long bolster and blocks

19 Inverted Lake

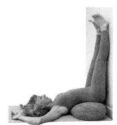

Hips on blankets or bolster, bottom ribs supported

Balancing the Pelvic Floor

1 Stand Tall

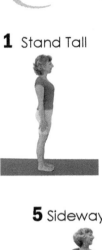

2 Sideways Lunge

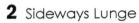
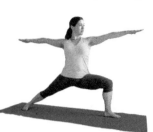

3 Stand Tall

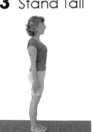

4 Forward Fold

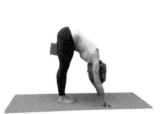

5 Sideways Lunge

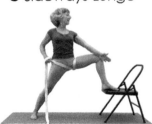

With a chair

6 Side Angle Pose

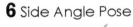
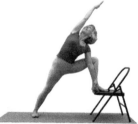

With a chair

7 Stand Tall

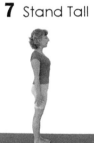

8 Forward Fold

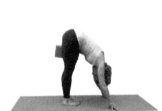

9 Standing Lunge

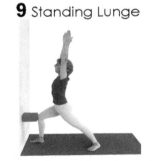

B. Knee holds block to wall

10 Stand Tall

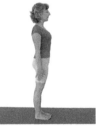
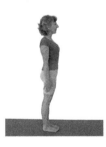

11 Straddle Forward Fold
concave back

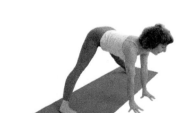

12 Straddle Forward Fold
rounded back

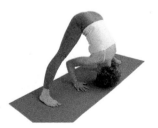

13 Chair Pose

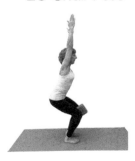

Basic Low Back Sequence

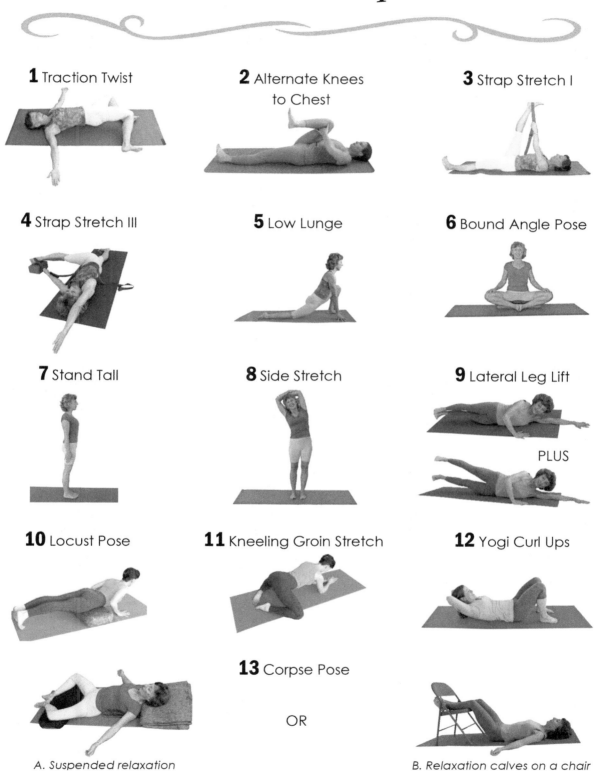

1 Traction Twist

2 Alternate Knees to Chest

3 Strap Stretch I

4 Strap Stretch III

5 Low Lunge

6 Bound Angle Pose

7 Stand Tall

8 Side Stretch

9 Lateral Leg Lift

PLUS

10 Locust Pose

11 Kneeling Groin Stretch

12 Yogi Curl Ups

13 Corpse Pose

OR

A. Suspended relaxation

B. Relaxation calves on a chair

Basic Neck & Shoulder Sequence

1 Basic Lying Twist
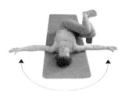

2 Yogi Curl Ups
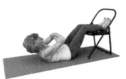

3 Supine Head Lift
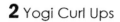

4 Half Fish Pose
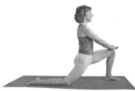

5 Traditional Cat/Cow

AND

6 Downward Facing Dog

A.

OR

B.
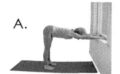

7 Low Lunge:
Hands on Knee

8 Elbows on the Chair
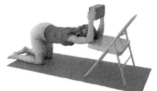

9 Eagle Arms Seated
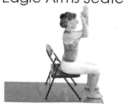

10 Cow's Head Arms
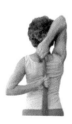

11 Sideways Chair Twist
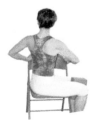

12 Door Chest Hang
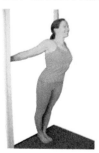

13 Corpse Pose
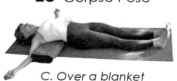

C. Over a blanket

Computer Recess

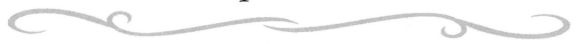

1 Traction Twist

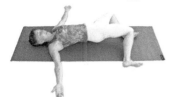

2 Pelvic Lift

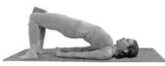

A. Hold block between knees

3 Basic Lying Twist

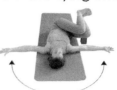

4 Yogi Curl Ups

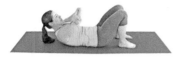

A. Hold elbows, up in center

AND

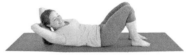

C. Curl up with twist

5 Supine Head Lift

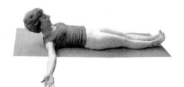

6 Half Fish Pose

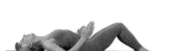

7 Open Twist in Chair

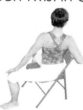

8 Reverse Plank

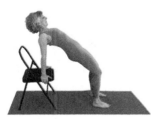

9 Downward Facing Dog

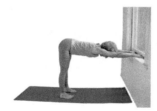

A. Hands on wall

OR

C. Feet on block at wall

10 Locust Pose

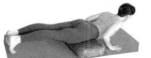

A. Across bolster, chest only lifts

OR

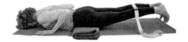

B. Belt mid-calf, legs only lift

11 Wide Leg Child's Pose

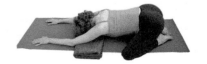

Leg Toning Sequence

1 Basic Lying Twist

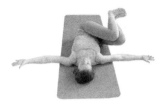

2 Traction Twist

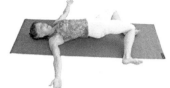

3 Alternating Knee Curl Ups

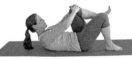

A. Bent knees

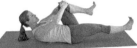

B. One leg extended

4 Yogi Curl Ups

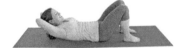

B. Arms behind head   *C. Shoulder toward opposite knee*

5 Yoga Leg Lifts

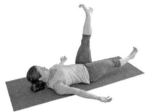

A. Lower alternate legs

6 Stand Tall

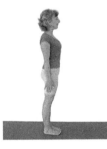

7 Sideways Lunge

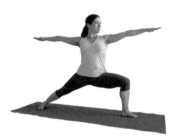

8 Standing Lunge

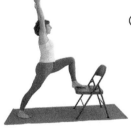

OR

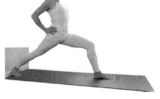

A. Foot on chair   *C. Rear heel at wall*

9 Split Leg Forward Fold

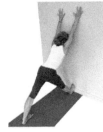

AND

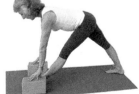

A. Hands on wall   *B. Hands on blocks*

10 Standing Scissor Twist

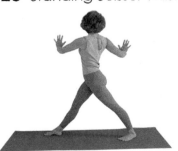

Leg Toning Sequence

11 Standing Chair Twist

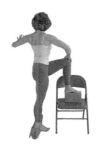

12 Standing Hand to Foot Pose

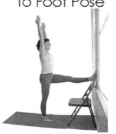

13 Standing Hand to Foot Pose and Twist

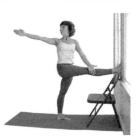

14 Straddle Forward Fold concave back

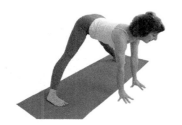

15 Straddle Forward Fold rounded back

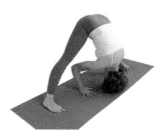

16 Pelvic Lift

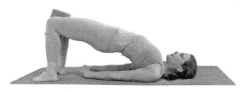

OR

A. Hold block between knees

B. Belt above knees

17 Corpse Pose

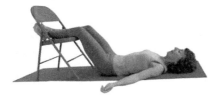

OR

Calves on a chair seat

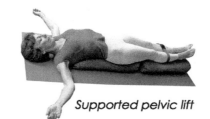

Supported pelvic lift

Progressive Abdominal Toning

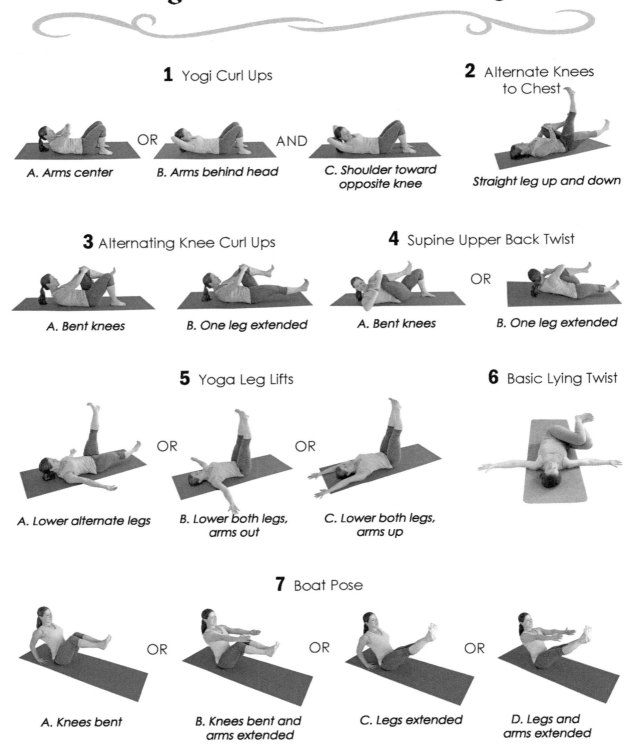

1 Yogi Curl Ups

A. Arms center   OR   B. Arms behind head   AND   C. Shoulder toward opposite knee

2 Alternate Knees to Chest

Straight leg up and down

3 Alternating Knee Curl Ups

A. Bent knees   B. One leg extended

4 Supine Upper Back Twist

A. Bent knees   OR   B. One leg extended

5 Yoga Leg Lifts

A. Lower alternate legs   OR   B. Lower both legs, arms out   OR   C. Lower both legs, arms up

6 Basic Lying Twist

7 Boat Pose

A. Knees bent   OR   B. Knees bent and arms extended   OR   C. Legs extended   OR   D. Legs and arms extended

Remember, this is NOT a sequence. Please choose poses according to your current needs and abilities.

Progressive Twists for Back Care

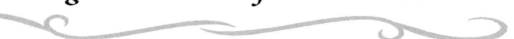

1 Traction Twist

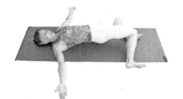

2 Basic Lying Twist

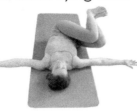

3 Yogi Curl Ups with a Twist

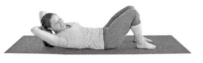

4 Supine Upper Back Twist

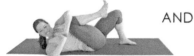 AND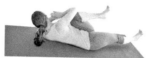

A. Bent knees   *B. One leg extended*

5 Sideways Chair Twist

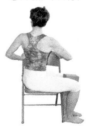

6 Open Chair Twist

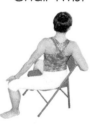

7 Standing Scissor Twist at Wall

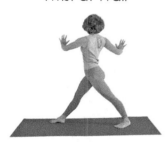

8 Standing Chair Twist

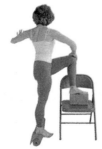

9 Standing Hand to Foot

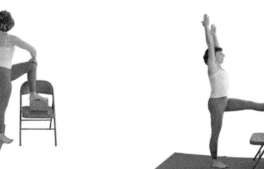

10 Standing Hand to Foot and Twist

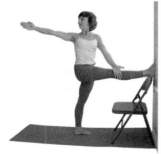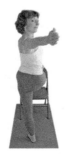

11 Prone Twist on a Bolster

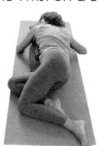

Progressive Spinal Extensions

1 Traction Strap Stretch I, II, III

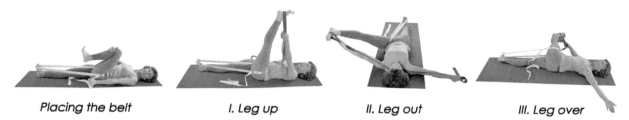

Placing the belt   *I. Leg up*   *II. Leg out*   *III. Leg over*

2 Pelvic Lifts   **3** Half Fish Pose

OR   OR

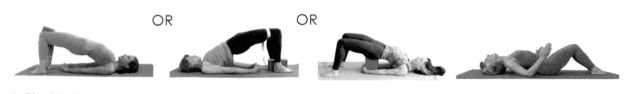

A. Block between knees   *B. Belt knees*   *C. Block under sacrum*

4 Lunges

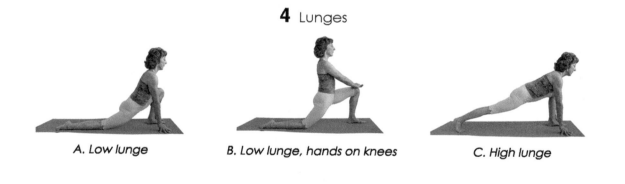

A. Low lunge   *B. Low lunge, hands on knees*   *C. High lunge*

5 Standing Lunge

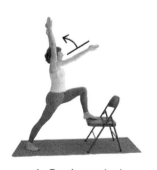
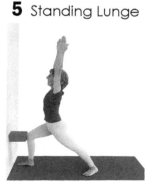
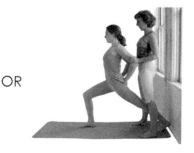

OR   OR

A. Foot on chair   *B. Knee holds block to wall*   *C. Rear heel at wall*

Progressive Spinal Extensions

6 Door Chest Hang

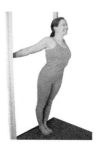

7 Reverse Plank with a Chair

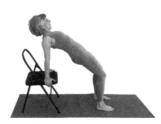

OR

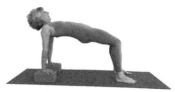

A. On a chair

B. Hands on blocks

8 Upward Facing Dog

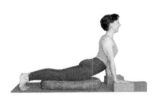

OR

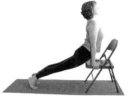

*A. Legs on bolster,
hands on blocks*

B. Hands on a chair

9 Downward Facing Dog

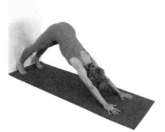

B. Hands and feet down

10 Locust Pose

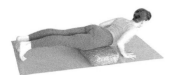

OR

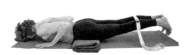

*A. Across bolster,
chest only lifts*

*B. Belt mid-calf,
legs only lift*

11 Wide Leg Child's Pose

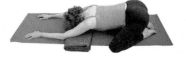

12 Pelvic Lift

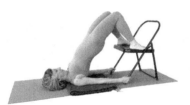

D. Feet in chair

13 Corpse Pose

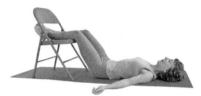

B. Calves on a chair seat

Sacral Un-Sticking Sequence

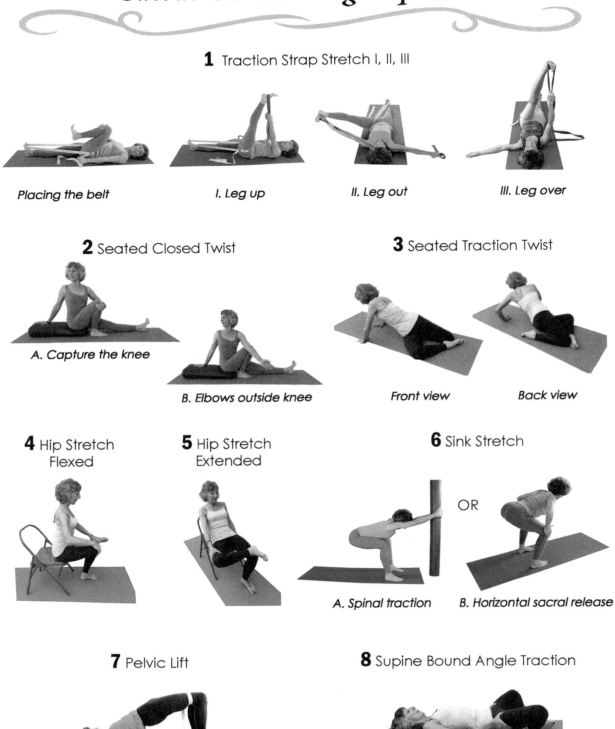

1 Traction Strap Stretch I, II, III

Placing the belt *I. Leg up* *II. Leg out* *III. Leg over*

2 Seated Closed Twist

A. Capture the knee

B. Elbows outside knee

3 Seated Traction Twist

Front view *Back view*

4 Hip Stretch Flexed

5 Hip Stretch Extended

6 Sink Stretch

OR

A. Spinal traction *B. Horizontal sacral release*

7 Pelvic Lift

B. Belt above knees

8 Supine Bound Angle Traction

Shoulder Release Sequence

1 Sideways
Chair Twist

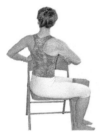

Block between knees

2 Open Twist
in Chair

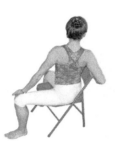

3 Eagle Arms
Seated

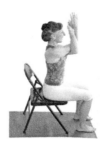

4 Closed Twist
in Chair

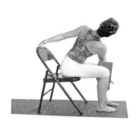

Block between knees

5 Half Cow's
Head Arms

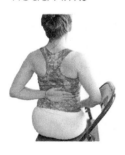

6 Upward Facing
Staff in Chair

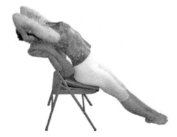

7 One Arm Sideways
Extension at Wall

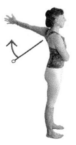

8 Upward Hands
Facing the Wall

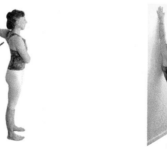

9 Both Arms
Extended Back

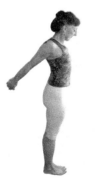

10 Bound
Finger Extension

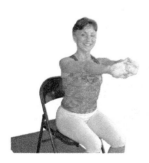

11 Reverse Wrist
Bend Seated

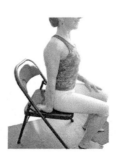

12 Forward Fold with
Head Support

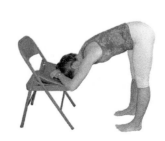

Shoulder Toning Sequence

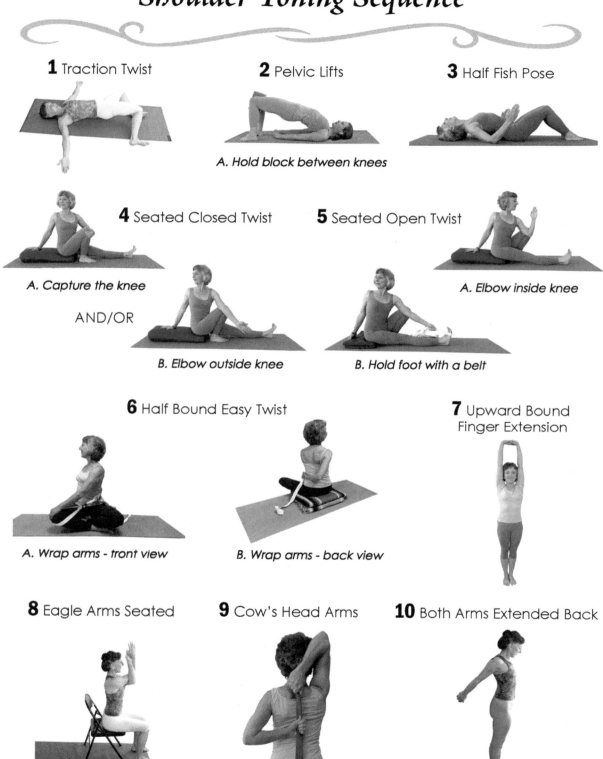

1 Traction Twist

2 Pelvic Lifts

A. Hold block between knees

3 Half Fish Pose

4 Seated Closed Twist

A. Capture the knee

AND/OR

B. Elbow outside knee

5 Seated Open Twist

A. Elbow inside knee

B. Hold foot with a belt

6 Half Bound Easy Twist

A. Wrap arms - front view

B. Wrap arms - back view

7 Upward Bound Finger Extension

8 Eagle Arms Seated

9 Cow's Head Arms

10 Both Arms Extended Back

Shoulder Toning Sequence

11 Sideways Wrist Stretch

12 Arms Overhead with a Pole

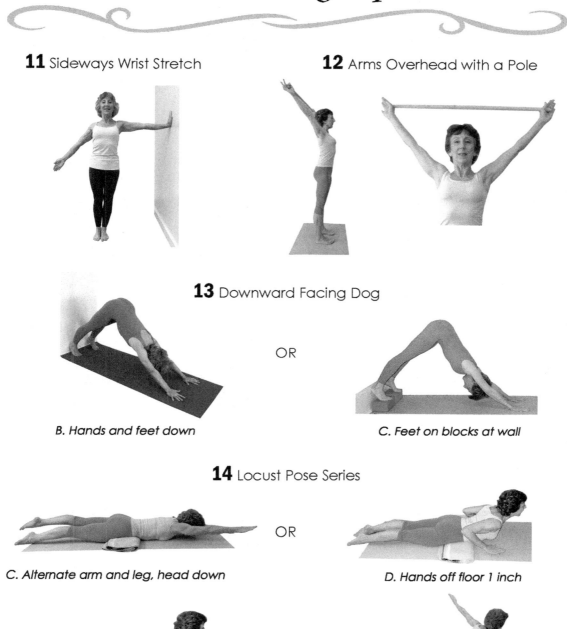

13 Downward Facing Dog

OR

B. Hands and feet down

C. Feet on blocks at wall

14 Locust Pose Series

OR

C. Alternate arm and leg, head down

D. Hands off floor 1 inch

OR

E. Arms extending back

F. Arms out to side, flying

Please choose one variation of the Locust Pose according to your current needs and abilities.

Shoulder Toning Sequence

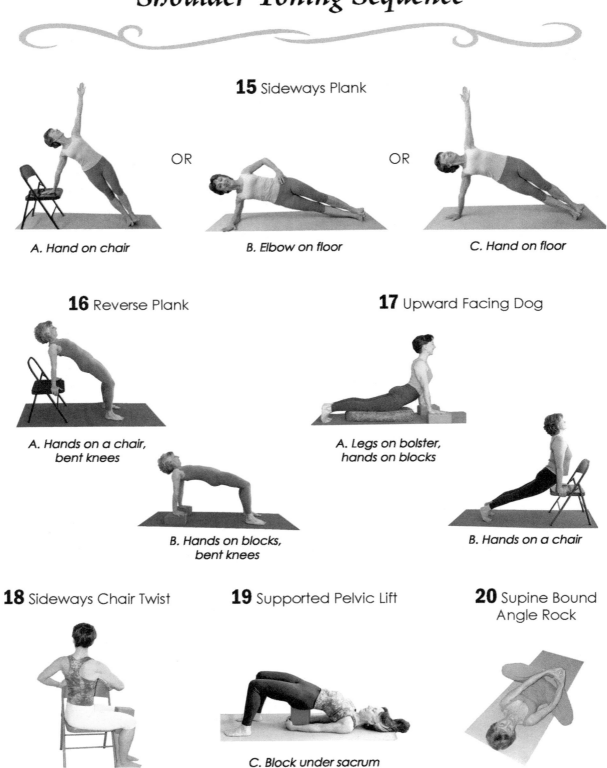

15 Sideways Plank

OR   OR

A. Hand on chair

B. Elbow on floor

C. Hand on floor

16 Reverse Plank

A. Hands on a chair, bent knees

B. Hands on blocks, bent knees

17 Upward Facing Dog

A. Legs on bolster, hands on blocks

B. Hands on a chair

18 Sideways Chair Twist

19 Supported Pelvic Lift

C. Block under sacrum

20 Supine Bound Angle Rock

First Level Shoulder Toning Sequence

1 Basic Lying Twist
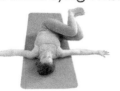

2 Traction Twist
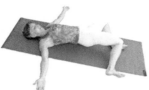

3 Pelvic Lifts
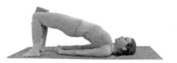

A. Hold block between knees

4 Half Fish Pose
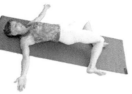

5 Seated Closed Twist
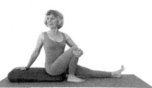

A. Capture the knee

6 Seated Open Twist
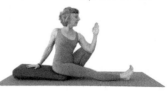

A. Elbow inside knee

7 Upward Bound Finger Extension
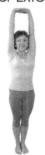

8 Eagle Arms Seated
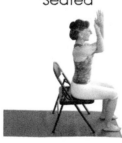

9 Cow's Head Arms
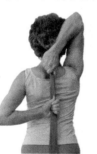

10 Both Arms Extended Back

11 Sideways Wrist Stretch
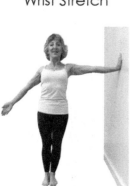

12 Arms Overhead with a Pole
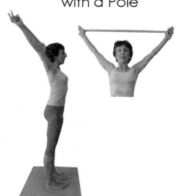

13 Locust Pose
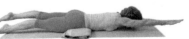

C. Alternate arm and leg

14 Downward Facing Dog
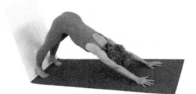

B. Hands and feet down

Second Level Shoulder Toning Sequence

1 Upward Bound Finger Extension

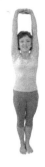

2 Eagle Arms Seated

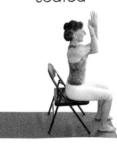

3 Both Arms Extended Back

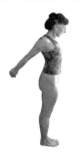

4 Arms Overhead with a Pole

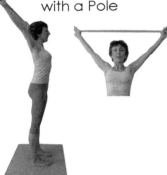

5 Downward Facing Dog

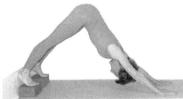

C. Feet on blocks at wall

6 Locust Pose

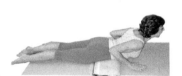

D. Hands off the floor 1 inch

7 Sideways Plank

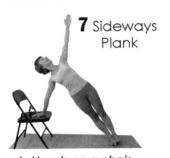

A. Hands on a chair

8 Reverse Plank

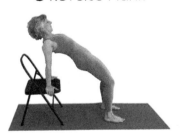

A. Hand on a chair

9 Upward Facing Dog

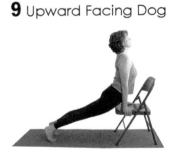

A. Hand on a chair

10 Downward Facing Dog

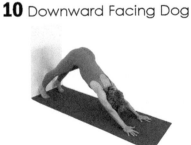

B. Hands and feet down

11 Sideways Chair Twist

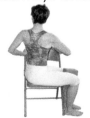

12 Pelvic Lift

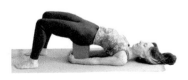

C. Block under sacrum

13 Supine Bound Angel Rock

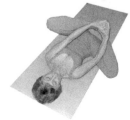

Third Level Shoulder Toning Sequence

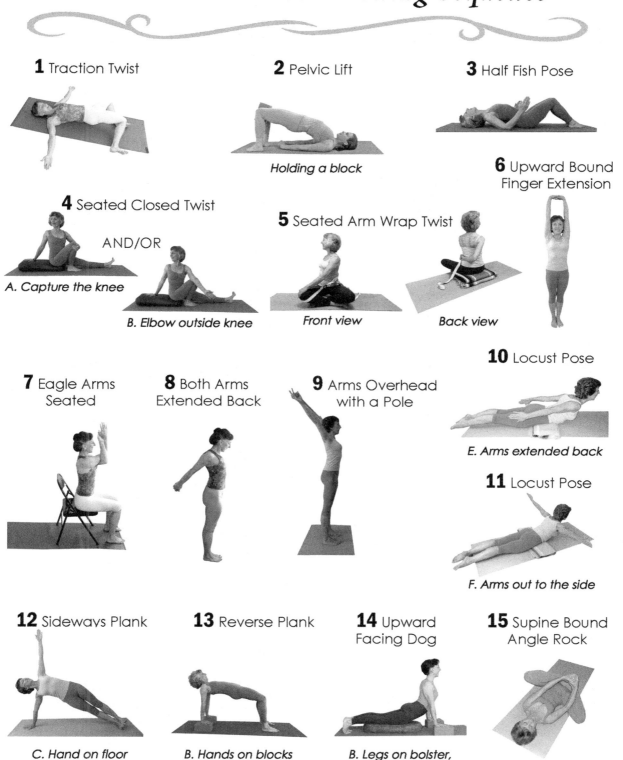

1 Traction Twist

2 Pelvic Lift

Holding a block

3 Half Fish Pose

6 Upward Bound Finger Extension

4 Seated Closed Twist

AND/OR

A. Capture the knee

B. Elbow outside knee

5 Seated Arm Wrap Twist

Front view

Back view

7 Eagle Arms Seated

8 Both Arms Extended Back

9 Arms Overhead with a Pole

10 Locust Pose

E. Arms extended back

11 Locust Pose

F. Arms out to the side

12 Sideways Plank

C. Hand on floor

13 Reverse Plank

B. Hands on blocks

14 Upward Facing Dog

B. Legs on bolster, hands on blocks

15 Supine Bound Angle Rock

Six Basic Restorative Poses

1 Reclined Bound Angle
with Full Support

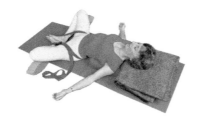

2 Supported Pelvic Lift

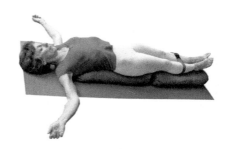

3 Prone Twist on Bolster

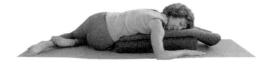

4 Sleeping Frog Prone on a Bolster

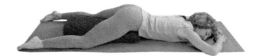

5 Inverted Lake Pose

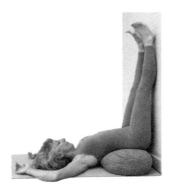

6 Corpse Pose

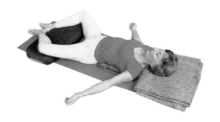

A. Suspended relaxation

Appendix

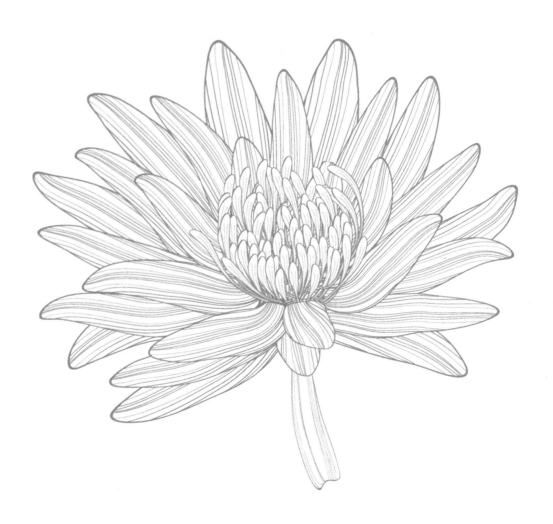

SOAP Chart

The word SOAP is an abbreviation used in a therapeutic context that stands for Subjective, Objective, Assessment and Plan. Hopefully by using this chart at the beginning of your practice and then 6–8 weeks later, you will begin to become more objective about your very subjective experience with back pain and have a way to track your improvement with the blessing of yoga.

Please mark the location and your perception of your back pain on the images below. Give each location a number from 1–10. Use the symbols in the key below to specify the type of pain.

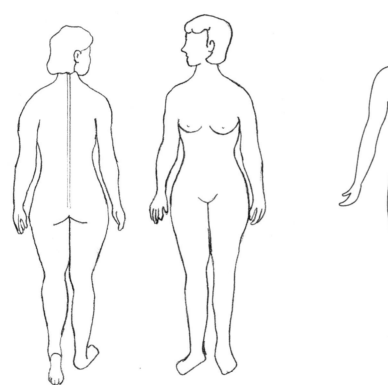

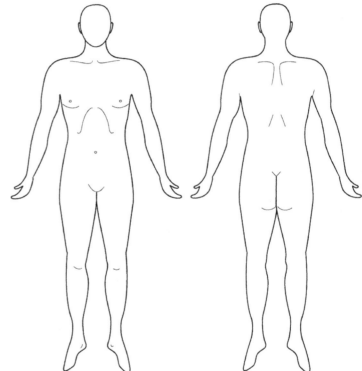

BEGINNING OF PRACTICE

SOAP Chart

After spending time with the recommended practices in this book for 6–8 weeks, access your progress by filling out this chart and comparing it to your first chart. You might also choose to make a copy of this page and re-access again after 6 months and again after 1 year.

Please mark the location and your perception of your back pain on the images below. Give each location a number from 1–10. Use the symbols in the key below to specify the type of pain.

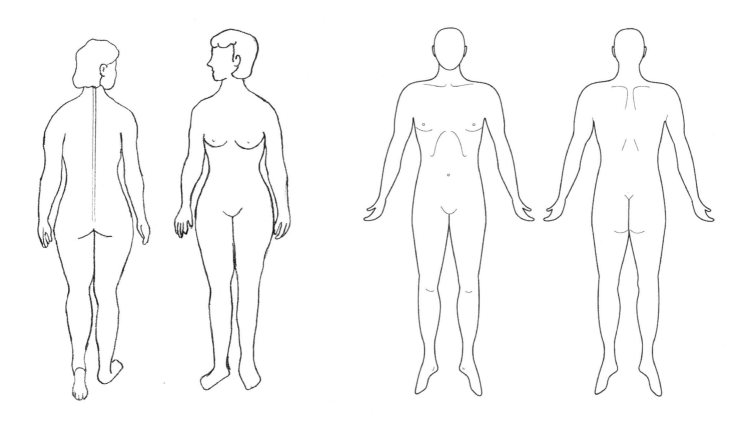

AFTER 6 WEEKS OF PRACTICE

Bibliography

Austin, Miriam. *Cool Yoga Tricks*. Ballantine Books, 2003

Calais-Germain, Blandine. *Anatomy of Movement*. Eastland Press, 1993.

Carrigan, Catherine. *What is Healing?* TotalFitness, 2013.

Couch, Jean. *The Runner's Yoga Book*. Rodmell Press, 1990.

Fishman, Loren, MD, and Carol Ardman. *Sciatica Solutions*. New York: W.W. Norton & Company, 2006.

Fishman, Loren, MD, and Carol Ardman. *Cure Back Pain with Yoga*. New York: W.W. Norton & Company, 2006.

Imrie, David, MD and Lu Barbuto. *The Back Power Program*. Wiley Science Editions, 2009.

Kabat-Zinn, Jon, PhD. *Full Catastrophe Living*. Bantam, 2013.

Mehta, Silva, and Shyam Metha. *Yoga The Iyengar Way*. Alfred A. Knopf, 1990.

Miller, Elise Browning. *Yoga For Scoliosis Work Book*. Spiral Bound, 2003.

Myers, Thomas W. *Anatomy Trains*. Churchill Livingstone, 2014.

Schatz, Mary Pullig, MD. *Back Care Basics*. Rodmell Press, 2000

Web Articles About Fascia

Barnes, John. F. "Therapeutic Insight: The Myofascial Release Perspective—Piezoelectric Transformation. "
https://www.massagemag.com/therapeutic-insight-the-myofascial-release-perspectivepiezoelectric-transformation-8009/

Integrative Soft-Tissue Release: "Sciatica Approach"
http://www.fascialrelease.com/blog/sciatica-approach

Anatomy Trains: "About Anatomy Trains"
https://www.anatomytrains.com/about-us/

Fascia Memory Project: "Fascia Memory Theory"
http://www.chalicebridge.com/FasciaMem-Pg6-Theory.html

National Institute of Neurological Disorders and Stroke: "Fascial Plasticity"
http://www.ninds.nih.gov/disorders/backpain/detail_backpain.htm#3102_10

Web Articles About Stress

Evidence-Based Complementary and Alternative Medicine: "Iyengar Yoga Increases Cardiac Parasympathetic Nervous Modulation Among Healthy Yoga Practitioners."
http://www.ncbi.nlm.nih.gov/pmc/articles/PMC2176143/

Pub Med.Gov: "Endorphin Levels in Cerebrospinal Fluid of Patients with Postoperative and Chronic Pain."
http://www.ncbi.nlm.nih.gov/pubmed/7091714

National Center for Complementary & Alternative Medicine: "Iyengar Yoga for Chronic Low-Back Pain Shows Promising Results."
http://nccam.nih.gov/research/results/spotlight/112409.htm?nav=cd

Ibid: "Yoga in Depth."
http://nccam.nih.gov/health/yoga/introduction.htm#thinking

National Institute of Neurological Disorders and Stroke: *Low Back Pain Fact Sheet*
http://www.ninds.nih.gov/disorders/backpain/detail_backpain.htm

Student Healing Stories

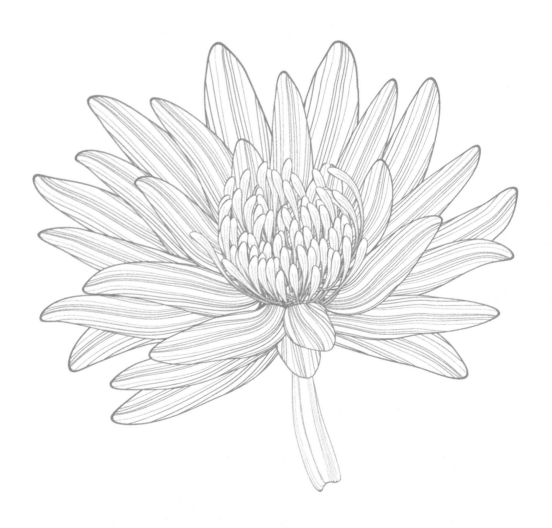

John's Back Story

When John first appeared for the eight-week yoga for back care series I was teaching, I was impressed by how tight he was all over his body. He was the classic muscle-bound male who over trained and never stretched. Not only the muscles but also the fascia in his body were clamped down. There was no room for his spine to extend. He started with a pain level of 8 out of 10, with three herniated/ bulging discs.

His yoga practice began with the first eight poses in the Basic Low Back Sequence, page 23. We then added some of the safe twisting poses practiced while seated or standing with a chair, along with the Alternate Low Back Sequence, pages 00-00. During the first three months, John needed to keep his hands on the wall for Downward Facing Dog, could lift only half way up in Pelvic Lift, and he focused primarily on Pose 16, Chair Twist standing at the wall to avoid negative pain. As time went on, he was able to work with all the variations of the Standing Lunge on page 79–80. For the next six months, his homework was to practice daily as much of the Hip Sequence as he could, along with Pose 14, Straddle Forward Fold Concave Back, page 100.

It took John nine months to experience complete freedom from back pain, which is to be expected with this deep level of neuromuscular change and healing. John's recovery is based on knowing which poses to focus on, patience, and a dedicated regular practice. Here's John summarizing his experience.

"The first time I remember injuring my back was around 1988. I bent over and felt a sharp pain in my back that just jerked me to the floor. The renowned spine surgeon I saw instructed me to do a stretch (basically a cobra pose) that lessened the pain. The MRI showed that I had torn the annulus between L4/L5 and had a bulge at L3/L4. I was sent to a physical therapist, who taught me a series of stretches and exercises that relieved the pain. I kept them up for a while, but after getting out of pain, slowly stopped doing them.

Over the next years, I ran three marathons and smaller distance races, never bothering to stretch much. I injured my back again several times. However, with rest and some exercises, the pain went away. Occasionally I would go to a yoga class with my wife. In 2012 and 2013, I did three U.S. Marine Corps Ultimate Challenge Mud Runs—a 10K run on a Marine base obstacle course. I forgot to mention I was 67! I am a competitor and always pushed myself and powered through exercises.

While preparing for the 2014 mud run, I was doing jumping lunges when suddenly I felt a sharp pain in my back. Tests confirmed a herniated disc at L3/L4 and large bulges in L4/L5 and L5/S1. My doctor recommended an epidural and physical therapy, but the pain persisted, and spinal surgery was discussed. I had learned, from my career in medical imaging and working with renowned spine surgeons, that operating should be the last resort. I also had seen many failed back operations. I was willing to do whatever was necessary to avoid an operation.

My wife, who had recently earned her 200-hour yoga teacher's certificate, had heard of a yoga teacher who focused on the back. She suggested I attend Lillah's workshop on Yoga for the Back. Lillah taught poses that focused on opening space in the spine and strengthening areas that affect the spine. I was not very good at the poses, didn't have much flexibility, and my core was weak. Lillah would scold me when I would attempt to "power" through a pose! She said I needed to learn how to relax and breathe while doing the pose. She also explained that after you injure your back, it would always be prone to injury. To keep my back strong, open, and free of injury, she stressed that I consistently practice the yoga poses and exercises to create length and space. When I completed the back series, I practiced several of the poses daily, and after six months my pain was gone completely. I continued to attend Lillah's class, refining the poses and practicing at home. Eventually I left the class but I continue to do several of the poses at home. Every once and awhile I forget my practice and do something that causes pain in my spine. I just immediately resume the poses she taught me and my back is relieved. I also at times return to her class for what I call a "refresher." I am 70 now, and as long as I continue to do the poses and exercises Lillah recommended, my back continues to stay strong and pain free. I am very grateful to Lillah for helping me avoid a spine operation, and for showing me how to relieve my pain and properly treat my back."

John J. Ariatti
Senior Consultant
Geoffrey Weiss & Associates

Shela's Hip Story

I am always delighted to see how well yoga works to help each practitioner rediscover and renew balance—physically as well as mentally. When Shela first came to my yoga class she had been out of shape and out of balance since her hip replacement surgery. Her surgery was performed from the front, which guided my choice of poses while she was healing. The physical abilities she has reclaimed are a delight to see. I will let her share her story here.

"I was 64 when I moved to Asheville in 2010, and it was pretty clear I was going to have to have hip surgery sooner than later. Like anyone in need of this surgery, my functionality was limited, and I was of feeling much older than I actually was chronologically. I had my surgery in June of the next year, as soon as I turned Medicare eligible. I recovered fairly quickly and was finally pain free. In November of that year, I started working with Lillah—thank you universe! In my first private session with her, she explained to me that after the type of surgery I had that there was a six- to nine-month window to regain full range of motion before the scar tissue and fascia harden, making a full recovery less then optimal. Applying yoga therapeutically throughout the healing process offered me a chance to regain full range of motion. Thank goodness I started working with Lillah within that six-month timeframe!

I have been taking yoga classes with Lillah and practicing consistently for a little over 2½ years now. The results I have experienced over time have been more than I could have hoped: my body is pain free—no back twinges like I used to experience fairly regularly, full range of motion, flexibility like I had in my thirties and forties, and the ability to take advantage of the wonderful lifestyle that Asheville, North Carolina, offers. I am now 68, and I can say I feel much younger and healthier than I could have expected at this age—much of this due to the regular practice of yoga. I really feel that most people would vastly benefit from a yoga practice, especially in our later years—and I highly recommend studying with Lillah!"

Shela Anmuth
Long Term Healthcare Insurance Specialist

Shela's first pose list:

1. Alternating Knee Curl Ups – Progressive Abdominal Toning, Pose 3, page 34.
2. Strap Stretch I and II – Alternate Low Back Sequence, Poses 6 and 7, page 39.
3. Bound Angle Pose – Basic Low Back Sequence, Pose 6, page 25.
4. Standing Lunge, Version A, front foot on chair – Progressive Spinal Extensions, Pose 5, page 79.
5. Downward Facing Dog Pose Version A, hands on ledge – Basic Neck and Shoulders Sequence, Pose 6, page 30.

Shela's second pose list added Strap Stretch III – Progressive Twists, Poses 5, 6, 7, 8, pages 64–65, and two standing poses to tone her legs and open her hamstrings from the Leg Toning Sequence – Split Leg Forward Fold, Pose 9, and Straddle Forward Fold, Pose 14, pages 98–100.

At the two and a half year mark, Shela's favorite poses that give her the most balance and freedom of movement include:

1. The Hip Sequence—particularly Traction Twists and Lunges, Poses 4, 7, and 8, pages 58 and 60.
2. Progressive Abdominal Toning—especially Alternate Knee to Chest with leg lifts, Pose 2, page 34.
3. Progressive Spinal Extensions — Downward Facing Dog, Pose 9 Version B, moving into Child's Pose, Pose 11, pages 82 and 83.
4. Leg Toning Sequence—Straddle Forward Fold, Pose 14, page 100.

Mary's Back Story

Mary Lenas had a sister who loved her and gave her three private lessons with me as a birthday present. Mary was a professional woman, age 46, who had been suffering with leg and back pain for over five years. She came to see me primarily for help with her back and knee pain. It seemed her right shin had been numb for some time. After going to physical therapy and acupuncture where she gained no relief, she chose to have a full neurological examination, and it was determined that she had nerve damage, which caused her shin to be numb. It seemed I was a last resort for some relief. Mary also suffered from fairly consistent migraines, had right sacroiliac pain, a shorter left leg, and mild scoliosis that affected both her hips and her shoulders.

Although I had no clear idea how things would unfold for her, I trusted the principles of yoga and knew that if I could help her create length and space particularly in her spine and hips, something would change for the better.

Mary lacked flexibility and was a bit fearful of activity because she didn't know how to discriminate between positive and negative pain. As she was young and healthy I started out boldly by teaching her the following series: Traction Strap Stretch I and III on page 75, Downward Facing Dog with hands on a chair, page 30, Chair Twist standing at the wall, page 65, and then a repeat of Downward Facing Dog. Mary practiced these poses at home daily for two weeks, and when she returned to see me, she had a 30 percent reduction in her right sacroiliac joint and knee pain.

In her next session, I taught her the full Hip Sequence and pelvic lifts to add to the above. I also added in poses to help her open her shoulders: Open Chair Twist, page 65, Eagle Arms, page 71, and Elbows on the chair, page 00. In her third session, I added standing poses from the Leg Toning Sequence to help integrate her hips with her spine: Standing Lunge, page 97, Sideways Lunge, page 96, and Straddle Forward Fold, page 100, ending with Inverted Lake Pose, page 49, for rest and integration. After three months of regular practice, not only was Mary's hip and knee pain gone, but her calf was no longer numb. By creating length and space, un-pinching the tubes, and establishing muscular balance—combined with consistent home practice—Mary was rewarded with greater than expected results.

One year later, Mary returned for another set of private lessons with a smile on her face, still enjoying life without hip or leg pain. This time we addressed the imbalance in her shoulders and chest caused by her scoliosis, which helped reduce the frequency of her migraines.

Sam's Shoulder Story

Sam was a small-framed man in his mid-thirties. He was born and raised in New Jersey and had participated in competitive weight lifting through high school and into his adult life.

His father, who knew me from social circles when I lived in Miami, asked Sam to come see me. As a young adult male, Sam's only job option was to be a night watchman where the physical demand was limited to his turning a key at each of his checkpoints. It seemed that Sam's hands kept going numb anytime he used his arms. He had already undergone one surgery on his right arm at the shoulder joint, shaving away some bone at the acromial-clavicular joint in order to open the nerve passage and thus relieve the numbness in his arm. The surgery had not helped. Sam had over trained. Not only were his muscles short and tight, but all the connective tissue in his arms was also bound up. Sam needed direction and encouragement.

We proceeded slowly using some of the arm positions from the Shoulder Release Sequence (see page 70). For Sam, even the simple movement of turning his palm to face out and then reaching back a short distance made his hand go numb. I helped him find his positive edge where he felt the sensation of stretch along his arm but stopped just before his hand went numb. I then guided him to hold the position for several deep relaxed breaths before releasing the pose to give the adhesions in the connective tissue a change to release and reorganize.

Sam and I met for a series of only three private lessons, but he was motivated, and committed himself to a home practice. So even though Sam practiced a sequence of only six yoga poses, he was able to create a profound change in his condition. After approximately eight weeks of practice, he returned to see me and happily reported that he had no numbness in his hands while freely moving his arms.

Sam's pose list:

1. Basic Twist – Progressive Twists, Pose 1, page 63
2. Traction Twist – Progressive Twists, Pose 2, page 63
3. Sideways Twist in a Chair – Shoulder Release Sequence, Pose 1, page 64
4. Closed Twist in a chair – Shoulder Release Sequence, Pose 4, page 72
5. Half Cow's Head Arms – Shoulder Release Sequence, Pose 5, page 72
6. One Arm Sideways Extension at the wall* – Shoulder Release Sequence, Pose 7, page 73
7. Elbows on the Chair – Basic Neck and Shoulder Sequence Pose 8, page 31

Sam started this pose with his hand at his hip and slowly inched his hand up the wall toward his waist and then higher.

My Personal Story

I started my yoga and healing journey many years ago with my first yoga teacher, David Carmos, in Boston, Massachusetts, in 1975. It seems destiny had a hand calling me forth in my study of yoga as a healing art. Through his example, David demonstrated the potential of yoga and diet to heal himself and others. He was my guide and inspiration as I embarked on my yoga journey. He quickened in me the desire and faith to pursue my own healing through yoga, which a few years later led me to the Iyengar method.

My study of Iyengar yoga, which began in 1978 in Miami, Florida, took me deeper into the art of yoga and how yoga had the potential to transform and heal.

After I had embarked on my teaching practice for about seven years, it became obvious to me that there were holes in my understanding. I was experiencing back, hip, and neck pain. Was it the yoga? Or was it me? I came to discover that it was me.

At the age of 16, I had sustained a fairly sizable impact in a horse accident, which rearranged the last 2 inches of my tailbone and caused me to suffer a bout of amnesia. The imbalance of my hip joints, pelvic floor, and sacrum that resulted from the accident caused, not only a short leg/long leg situation, but also torsion in my spine that affected my neck and shoulders, creating a scoliosis. Needless to say, I was beginning to experience back pain in more ways than one. So the more I tried to progress my practice into the advanced yoga postures, the more trouble I encountered.

Only one of my Iyengar teachers ever questioned me about my difficulties: her name was Felicity Green. She had been an occupational therapist before she was a yoga teacher, so she had a perspective on how the body functions that others did not. She had also recovered from several joint limitations herself. I related well to her perspective because I was also trained in anatomy and physiology as a licensed massage therapist. She helped me on several occasions to unravel my yoga practice in order to find pain relief.

It was a slow process of trial and error as I worked to put together an understanding of my body, how it functions, and how to sustain relief by adjusting my practice and my poses. My hip pain would travel; sometimes it was my left hip and sometimes my right. I can remember the year that my right hip ached almost constantly for six to nine months. It was embarrassing as I got up from a chair or the floor and had to hobble across the room before I could stand straight. It was through a combination of studying with the Iyengars in the U.S. and India, Felicity's insightful guidance, and the adjustment of my yoga practice over time, that I was able to rebalance my body and diminish the intensity of the pain.

Yoga has always been the healing force in my life. Over and over again when I returned to my mat I would find a way to relieve my discomfort and find ease.

There is one other challenging memory worth mentioning because it demonstrates the mind-body condition. For several months I lived with knife-like pain in the front of my deltoid muscles in my upper arms. I was experiencing a great deal of stress at the time and it seems that my shoulders were where the stress landed. Again, healing required changing my yoga practice. I repeated simple poses over and over until the neuromuscular and facial systems were again realigned and rebalanced, returning to me ease of movement and gratitude for the practice of yoga. During the process, the yoga also helped me to address the emotional components of my stress. Through good attention and an understanding of alignment and function, I was able to get to know the map of my body and what different sensations indicated, which allowed me to choose the best yoga poses to re-create balance and freedom.

It is my sincere hope and intention that the ideas about our bodies and the understanding of the poses I share in this book will contribute to your self-knowledge and healing journey. May you come to own your yoga practice. And may yoga bring you back to balance again and again, keep you free from pain, and help you to live a satisfying life.

Namaste, Lillah

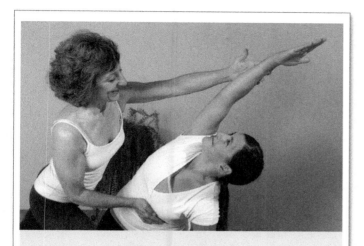

"*Lillah has both the knowledge and the passion to fulfill her mission of helping others on the path towards Dharma, the very reason for the practice of yoga. I recommend Lillah with all my heart.*"

—Aadil Palkhivala
Purna Yoga founder and author of *Fire of Love*

Two Companion DVDs

60–90 min. of instruction & guided practice, reference card included. DVDs Retail: $14.95 each

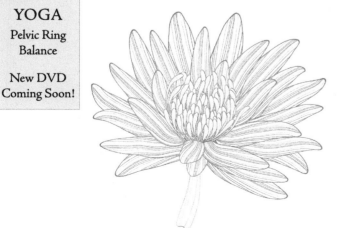

Yoga: Your Freedom from Back Pain
ISBN: DVD – 0964383519

Yoga: Relief from Neck & Shoulder Pain
ISBN: DVD – 0964383586

YOGA
Pelvic Ring
Balance

New DVD
Coming Soon!

Lillah A. Schwartz

Known as "the queen of alignment," yoga instructor, teacher trainer, and author Lillah Schwartz has studied with yoga experts such as B.K.S. Iyengar, Aadil Palkhivala, Eric Small, Matthew Sanford, and others.

She pioneered the Iyengar method in North Carolina from 1981, led the way to establishing Asheville as a yoga destination, and held an Iyengar teaching certificate from 1985–2009.

Lillah is well known for her excellence in the therapeutic applications of yoga based on 35 years of experience. Her Healing Our Backs with Yoga™ teaching program brings the science and spirit of yoga to hundreds of people each year, who have connected with their healing potential, overcome their pain, and improved their functional ability with her guidance. Her program is a registered yoga therapy course with IAYT. Founded on this program she has developed a book of the same name.

Through her popular DVDs, "Yoga: Your Freedom from Back Pain" and "Yoga: Relief from Neck and Shoulder Pain," Lillah brings the essence of dynamic alignment and yoga wisdom home in a practical, safe, and unique way. Recommended by Dr. Andrew Weil, *Prevention Magazine*, and *Yoga Journal*, these long-selling DVDs were called "an excellent resource for beginning yoga enthusiasts," by *Booklist*.

Lillah's weekly classes and individual yoga therapy sessions offer students the opportunity to deepen their practice and heal from injury. In addition, students experience an invitation to transformation during her yearly 200-hour and unique 300/500-hour Transformation Yoga Teacher Training programs.

Visit her website and blog...

at YogawithLillah.com for free videos and yoga tips; to purchase copies of her DVDs; schedule a private online session; or invite Lillah to your studio to teach a customized weekend or the popular Healing Our Backs with Yoga™ CE Therapy course.

CPSIA information can be obtained
at www.ICGtesting.com
Printed in the USA
LVOW06s0250100816
499728LV00016B/23/P